The Natural Glamour

The Ayurveda Beauty Book

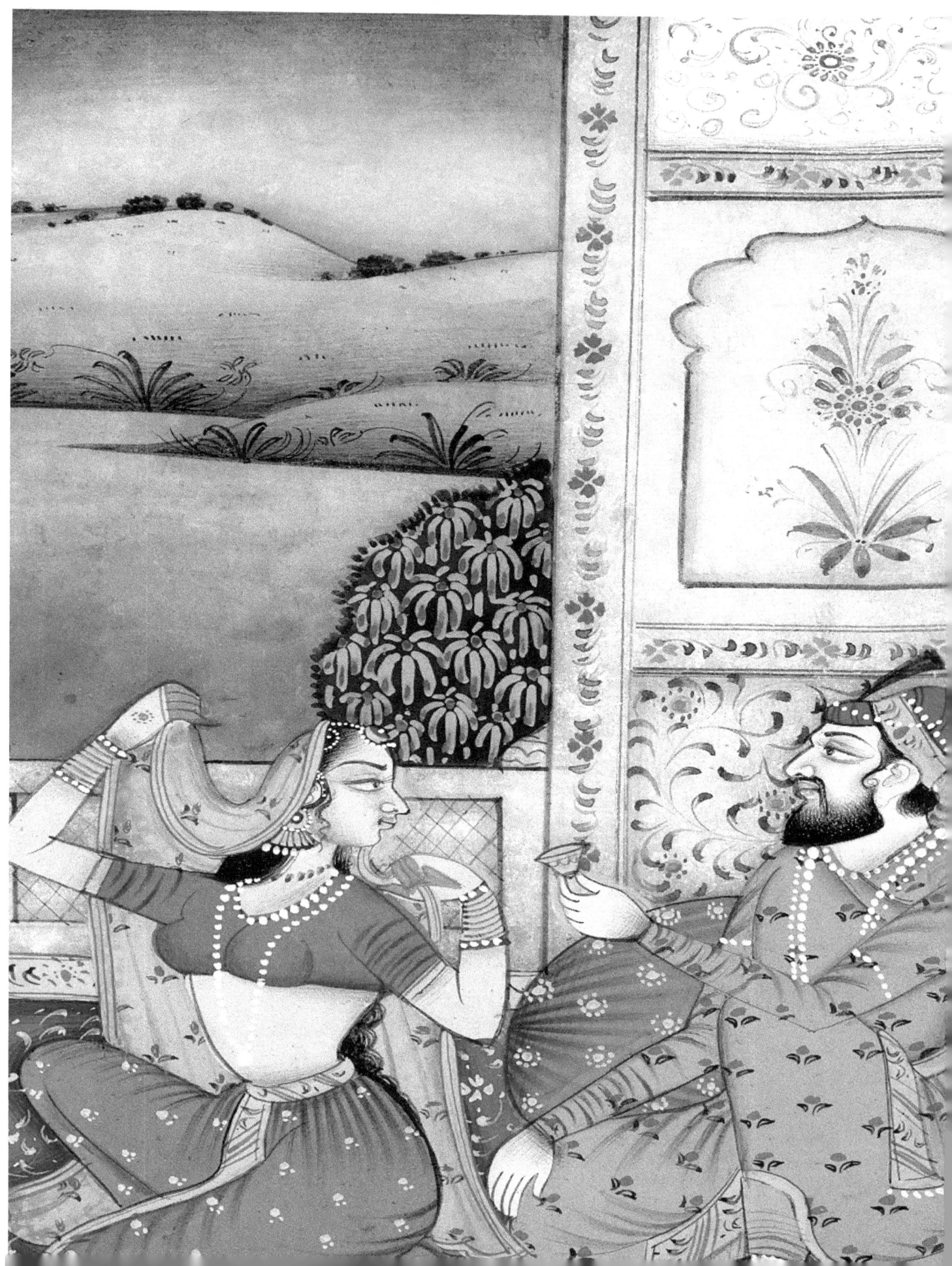

Dr. Vinod Verma

The Natural Glamour

The Ayurveda Beauty Book

Gayatri Books International

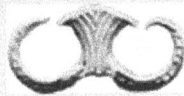

The information provided in this book is not intended to replace the services of a physician. Suggestions for a healthy way of living to have a better appearance and strength with Ayurvedic life-style and some external applications to enhance radiance are given in this book for the purpose of self-help and education. The author and the publisher are in no way responsible for any medical claims regarding the material presented in this book. Commercial use of methods and remedies suggested in this book requires the prior permission from the author. For more information, write to the author directly or in care of the publisher.

This book is also published in German in 2003 by Nymphenberger, Munich and Spanish in 2012

Published by Gayatri Books International, Himalayan Centre, Village Astal, Dunda, Uttarkashi-249151 (Uttarakhanda), India. Any legal matters will be handled in the jurisdiction of this address.

Translation rights are held by the author. Write to her at drvinodverma@dataone.in or ayurvedavv@yahoo.com or through the publisher: gayatribooks@yahoo.de.

Visit Dr. Vinod Verma at www.ayurvedavv.com to find out about her other publications, seminars, lectures and consultations. Look for more information on the last pages of the book.

Consultant editors: Kiran Sahni, Mohit Joshi

Cover design and photographs by the author

Photographs and art works: Author's personal collection

ISBN: 81-89514-28-8

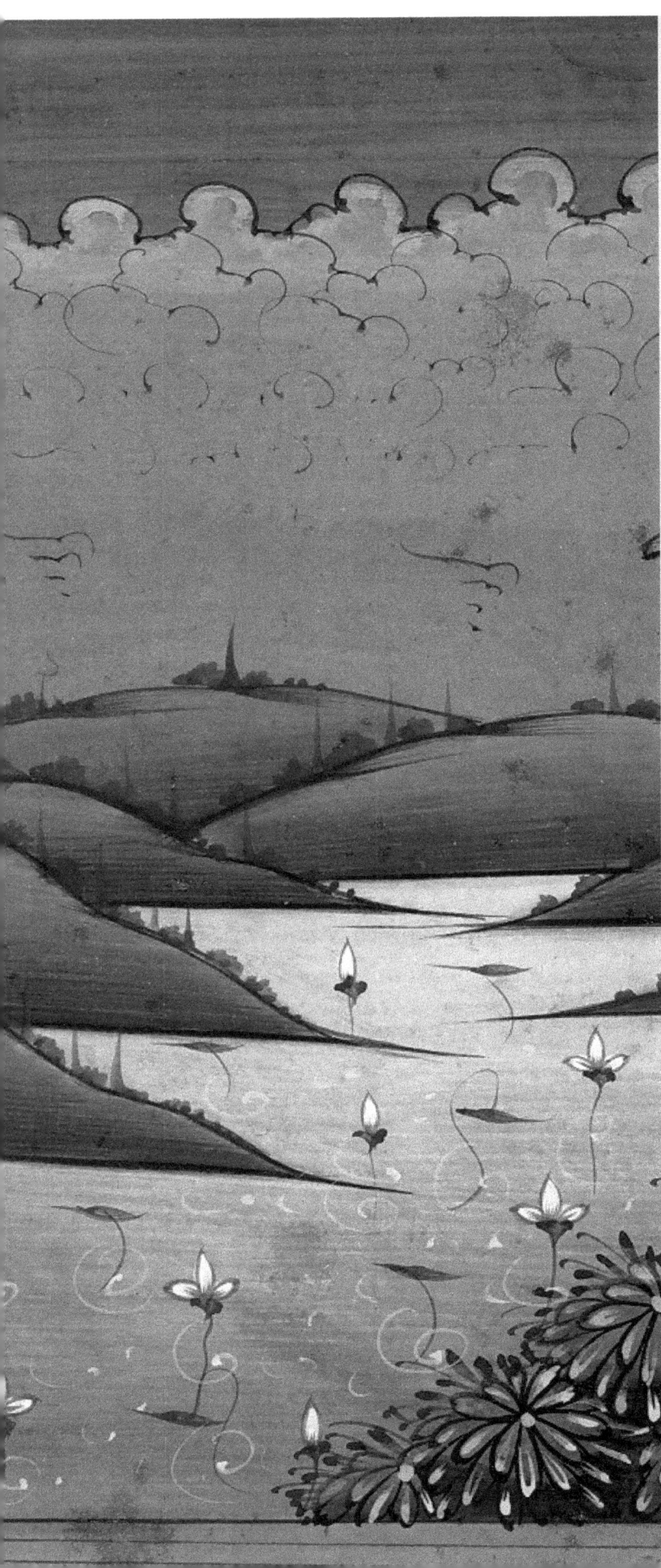

Dedication

This book is dedicated to the strength of the Himalayas, the beauty of the Bhagirathi (the upper Ganga in the Himalayas) and the splendour of the sun.

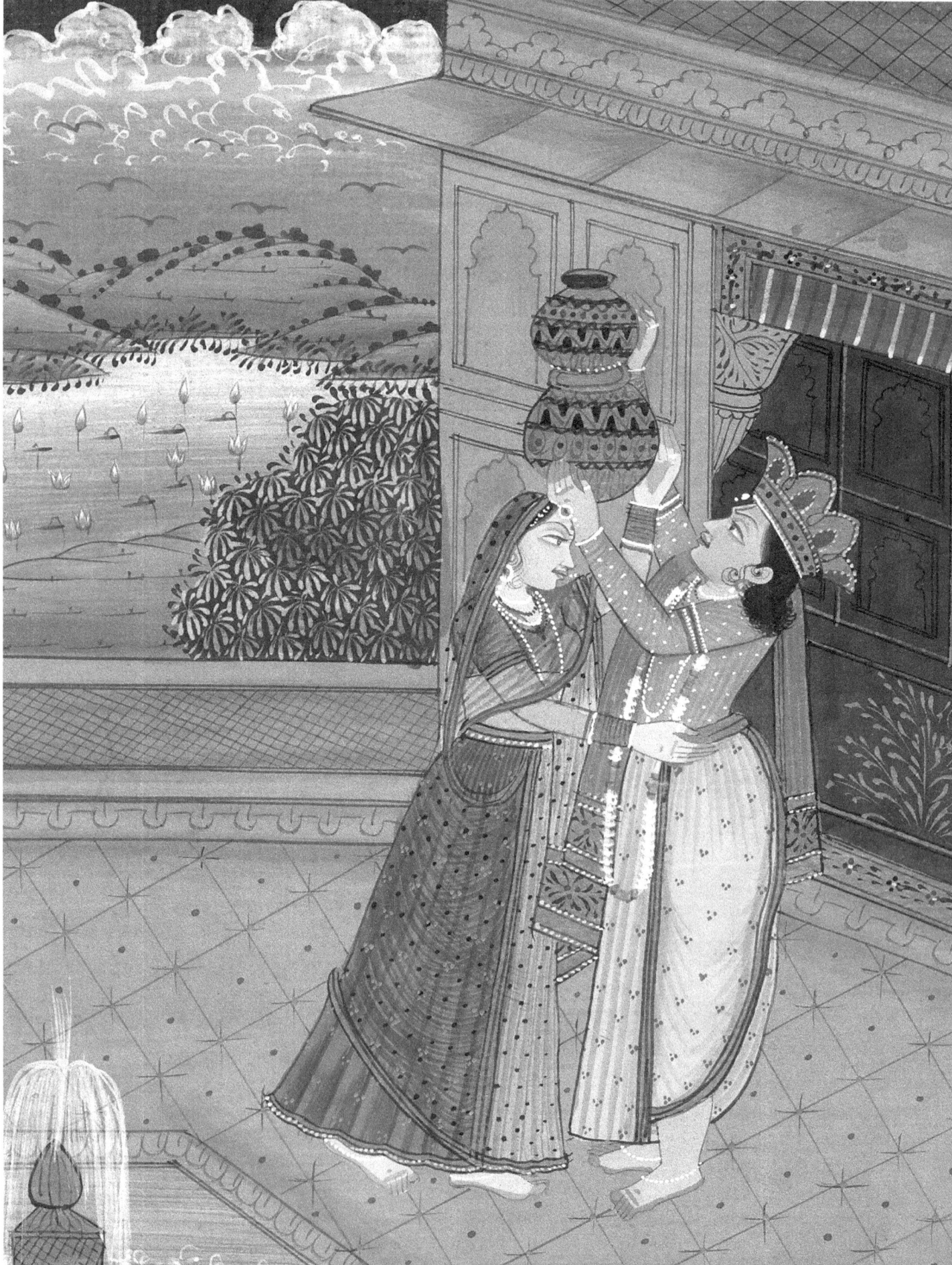

Contents

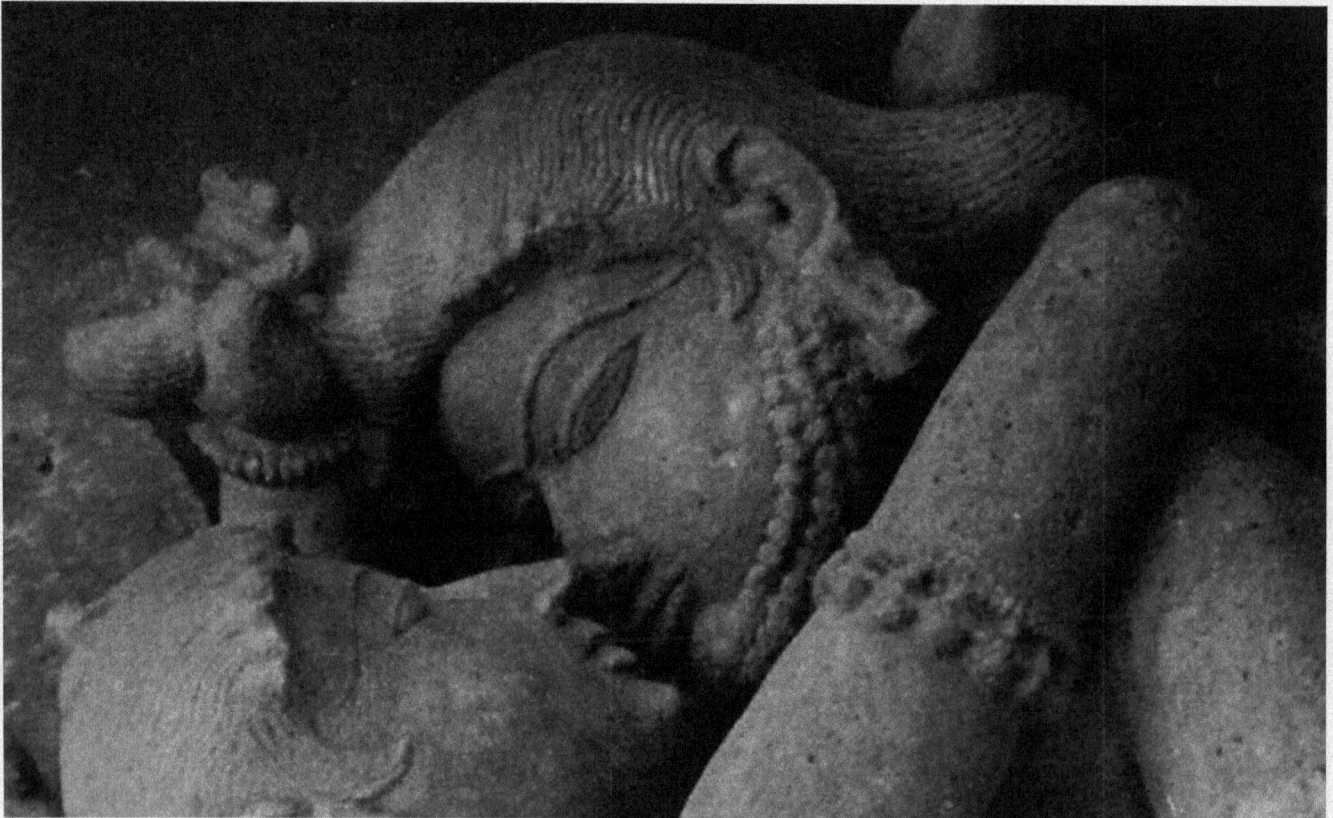

Preface

Millions are invested all over the world to make beauty products, and people, especially women, spend a fortune to either enhance their beauty or to cover up what is not beautiful. It is a natural desire to beautify oneself but unfortunately, it is poorly understood that an attractive appearance, glowing skin and charm are directly related to one's mental and physical health. There are numerous advertisements on the television the world over for products, which promise you beautiful skin, remove pimples, bags under the eyes, and so on. Yet, most actors and actresses have bad skin and one sees pimples on their faces in close ups. According to the Vedic tradition, our beauty is from birth and is the result of our good karma but we should maintain it with our present karma. Obviously, in the film and television industry, they are quite unaware of holistic Ayurvedic methods to maintain and enhance glamour by purifying the body internally. Your pimples are not the problem of your skin but of your entire body. Only a blood purifier will make you get rid of them and not merely the external application of some creams. Your blood with various toxic impurities will not only give you pimples but also other ailments in course of time. Thus, beauty is both, inner and outer and the 'inner' reflects on your appearance. Health and beauty are interrelated and not being sick does not mean that you are healthy. A condition of equilibrium that gives you the optimum level of mental and physical vitality and immunity will automatically makes you look attractive and radiant. This book tells you what all to do to get the inner balance and outer beauty and glamour.

Many years ago, when I was a student in Paris, a Canadian friend of ours commented about one of our South Indian friends that she has a kind of beauty western women are aspiring for. She explained that she had a naturally shining skin which women in the West try to acquire with special kinds of makeup, which would not look like makeup. Young people should normally have a glowing complexion and that is still very true for our village population. Once I heard my mother and some other elderly persons of the family saying that these days young persons do not have the *roop* as they used to have during their times. What is this *roop*? *Roop* is not beauty but a sense of harmony and glamour along with radiance. Radiance is called *shree* in Sanskrit. Roop is the strength and glow of youth that oozes out. In Ayurveda, it is called *ojas*. Ojas is the vitality and vigour of life as well as the capacity to protect and defend life from external attacks, which we call immunity. But in the present context, it is taken in the sense of radiance that vitality gives rise to.

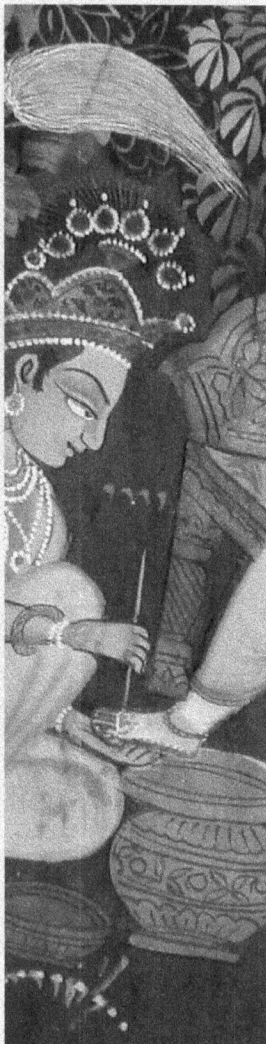

It is indeed very true that young people in the cities no longer have glow and charm on their faces. Their health is also not good and many of them have skin problems like acne, which are the result of imbalance in body's energy and impurities in the blood.

The purpose of this book is to help you attain *roop* and maintain a youthful appearance with various external applications, through nutrition and lifestyle, and inner purification of the body. There are simple methods to take care of yourself and you will notice a tremendous difference. Television ads tell you very easy ways to make you beautiful and radiant by using certain creams and oils and other treatments. Actually a dull complexion, rough skin and pimples can be treated with external applications only to a very limited extent. You need to go to the root of the problem and eradicate it. According to Ayurveda, when the three energies of your body are not in balance, you are in an unhealthy state. Your external appearance is nothing but the reflection of your internal state. Besides the energies of the body, your mental state plays a great role in your appearance.

Everyone, men, women and children want to look healthy and beautiful. The books on beauty are generally written for women or they are considered exclusively for women. Men, particularly in the West are usually conditioned not to beautify themselves. However, in Indian tradition, during various ceremonies before marriage, man and woman are given similar Ayurvedic beauty treatments. I am going to give you in this book the general Ayurvedic and yogic wisdom to enhance your health and to obtain a radiant look. These methods are also meant to be used as an investment for your old age by which I do not mean clichés like how to get rid of wrinkles, and so on.

In this holistic book on beauty, we will deal with your physical and mental state, as well as the radiations your inner self exuberates. There are also some breathing methods (pranayama) and concentration practices (japa) for your health and external appearance.

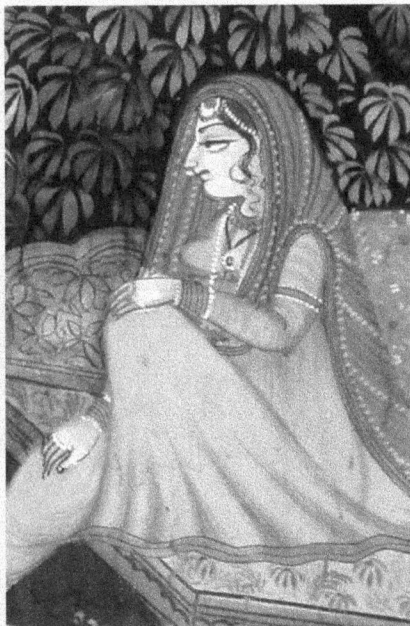

The first chapter deals with the holistic way of life, which is essential for attaining a beautiful and attractive look in a natural way. The second chapter explains the relationship of your inner being to your outer appearance. The third chapter deals with the various external methods to acquire an attractive look as well as some internal purification to eradicate the causes that spoil your roop and shree. The fourth chapter demonstrates the use of various oil massages, oil treatments, anointing and fomentation therapy you can do on your own to attain strength and beauty. These not only enhance your external appearance but they also provide you with physical strength and mental balance. Those who have hectic lifestyles and stressful jobs will get special relief from these easy-to-do self-treatments. The fifth chapter is on nutrition and its effect on your health and appearance. The sixth chapter has some specific yogic methods and yogic dance (*yoga nritya*) to make you flexible and to attain proper blood circulation in each part of your body to give you a charming look and glowing complexion. Yoga nritya is the result of my latest research and has proved very fruitful in relaxing the mind and beautifying the appearance. The seventh chapter deals with spirituality for initiating you to develop a relationship with time (*kala*) and various cosmic bodies in order to enhance your radiance. There are also methods to acquire energy from various cosmic bodies like the radiance of the sun, the poise and wisdom of moon and dignity of the stars. The eighth chapter contains a glossary of the products and other things that I have referred to in the book, their description and availability.

Even if you do not use all the suggestions given in this book, it will bring you still lot of benefit. Reading this book will at least make you aware of the various dimensions of your lifestyle that affect your appearance, as well as health.

Vinod Verma
July, 2002
www.ayurvedavv.com
ayurvedavv@yahoo.com

Present Edition: January 2014

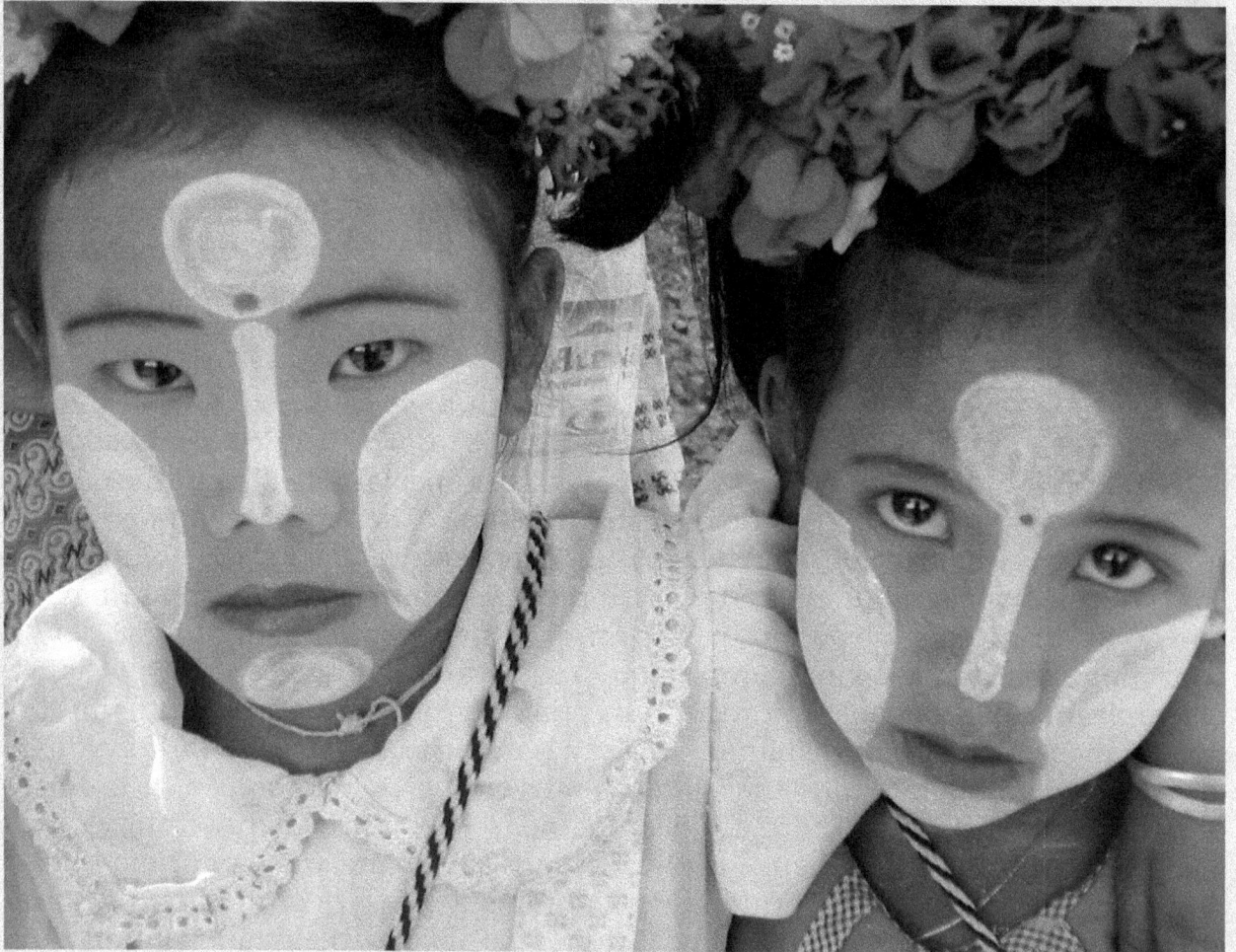

1
The State of Health and Non-health

Healthy body with Shree and Roop

'Shree'* in Sanskrit means the energy we exuberate. Some people in the West call it aura or a good aura. Shree is our radiance. 'Roop' is the harmony and glamour along with the radiance. Roop is supported by shree as shree enhances the roop. Shree is the energy that is behind the physical form. It reflects our inner harmony and peace. For example a good looking and charming person, when afraid or under any other kind of extreme mental pressure appears without any radiance. In Sanskrit, it is called shreeheen (without shree). The synonym of shree is Kanti which literally means radiation.

Health and beauty are inseparable from each other. Health does not only mean a state of physical well being free of ailments. Health is your well being in totality. It also includes your mental disposition. A person with lack of self-confidence, easily afraid and nervous cannot be stated as healthy. Not only this person loses Shree or Kanti, but a nervous state of mind and allied characteristics lead to series of disorders. Physical health in Ayurveda is related to mental health as well as to familial and social harmony. Personal effort plays an important role and maintaining health is each individual's primary responsibility. That is what we all owe to our existence or being.

The dynamic body

As a normal and healthy person, you notice that you feel differently each day. There are some days when you feel dynamic and full of energy and there are other days when you feel more or less tired. There are days when you feel very positive and bright and there are other days when you feel dull and do not like to take any initiative. Sometimes you feel easily irritated and angry and ask yourself- 'What is wrong with me?' There are times when you think that you are not sick but you feel strange and rather weak. In other words, you have subjective symptoms of being unwell. These are contrary to objective symptoms. Objective symptoms are either measurable like fever or blood

---

* The word 'Shree' is also used as a prefix before the male names.

13

pressure, and so on, or they show concrete indicators like cold, cough or any kind of pain or burning sensations, etc.

The ups and downs in our state of health indicate that our body is a dynamic and ever changing system like the rest of the cosmos. In fact, we are a tiny bit in the infinite cosmos and fundamentally everything that exists functions in a similar manner. The whole cosmos is a bigger system whereas our body is a smaller system or a subsystem in the universe.

Dynamic body in the dynamic cosmos

In this cosmos, everything is interconnected and interdependent. The causative factor of the basic cosmic unity is the common constituent of all that exists. The five elements or mahabhutas are responsible for all that exists. These are ether (space), air, fire, water and earth. Without space nothing can exist. It is the primary factor. In space there is air. Fire needs both air and space to exist. The fourth element, water, is dependent on its existence on the previous three elements. Water has also the fire element. Think of the ice age and how everything came to existence after that. The earth is the fifth element and heaviest of all. It needs all the other four elements for its existence. Earth is most complete and heaviest of all the elements.

As we observe each day, the five elements in the cosmos are dynamic and well coordinated and form a perfect system. The sun brings us warmth and light each day and the darkness of the night is beautified with stars and the changing phases of the moon. There are clouds, rains, snow, and rivers which gush towards their destination. From the dynamism of the five elements, seeds become sprouts; trees lose their leaves and get new ones. The living being from both plant and animal world die and new life comes to being. There is no still moment in this dynamic cosmos and change is another name for time. Nothing is lost and there is constant transformation.

Like the cosmos, an individual living system is also perfect and dynamic. It is a part of the cosmos and likewise it is constituted of the five fundamental elements. But the elements in a living system are present in the form of three energies or doshas in order to perform all the functions of this particular system. To perform all the mental and physical functions of the body, the three energies coordinate with each other and make a perfect system. The body has further smaller systems or organisms, which perform their individual functions, and the three energies also coordinate these functions. These energies are called vata, pitta and kapha in Ayurveda and each has characteristics of the elements they are derived from.

The three principal energies of the body- vata, pitta and kapha

Vata is constituted from elements ether and air and its functions are related to these two elements. Ether or space is omnipresent and air is mobile. The functions related to movements as well as to space are performed by vata.

> **Vata** is responsible for entire body movements, blood circulation, respiration, excretion, speech, sensations, touch, hearing, feelings like fear, anxiety, grief, enthusiasm etc., natural urges, formation of foetus, sexual act and retention.

Fire constitutes the pitta energy of the body and thus pitta is body's fire or *agni*. When we use the word agni in Ayurveda, it pertains to everything related to digestion and assimilation. Agni in Ayurvedic terminology is a part of pitta but pitta has also some other functions.

> **Pitta** is responsible for vision, hunger, thirst, heat regulation, softness, lustre, cheerfulness, intellect and sexual vigour.

Kapha forms the solid part of the body and is responsible for the formation of new cells. Our body constantly needs new cells. We need various secretions in the body. Kapha is active during childhood for the growth of a baby. The inner lining of the digestive system and uterus is made of epithelial and these are constantly renewed.

> **Kapha** constitutes all the solid structure of the body and is responsible for binding different body organs together. It gives rise to firmness and heaviness to the body and is responsible for sexual potency, strength, forbearance and restraint.

Individual health and cosmic balance

Both body and cosmos are dynamic and they have the same fundamental constituents— the five elements. Just as we need the equilibrium of five elements in the cosmos for an order and harmony in the cosmic system, similarly, for good health, we need a balance of these elements, which constitute our body in the form of three energies. To imagine five elements in the body in the form of vata, pitta and kapha may sound abstract to you at this stage. It is easier to comprehend the system of three energies in the body and their equilibrium if we first understand how the five elements maintain the cosmic equilibrium and what happens when this equilibrium is disturbed.

Imagine a calm day when it is neither too hot nor too cold. The wind is blowing gently and there is a perfect ratio of humidity in the air. Everything seems serene and calm and you feel good in this kind of atmosphere. Imagine another day with very rough winds blowing. They uproot trees and destroy other things. If you are living on the bank of a river like me, there is a danger of flood from the fallen trees. First of all, the element wind was not in equilibrium. It disturbed the element earth and uprooted the trees. The trees were no longer where they should have been. Thus, the harsh winds disturb the element space. Flood disturbs the element water as it enters into the fields and destroys the crops. Once again, the element earth is disturbed. Thus we see that when one of the elements in nature does not function properly, the whole system is disturbed. Similarly, for good health, glowing complexion and good skin, the three energies or dosha of the body, made from five elements, should perform their functions in harmony with each other. If one of the energies is disturbed, we step into a state of imbalance and ill health.

We can also take other examples from nature. When the summer is too hot or it does not rain and there is drought, or there are accidents with the life-giving fire or there are floods or earthquakes, there is destruction. Similarly, when we do not maintain the equilibrium of the five elements in our system, there are disturbances and ill health. In other words, our system is built the same way as nature. If we go against nature, eat too much or too little or too frequently or do not sleep during the night or sleep during the day and do not care to go to the toilet on time, and so on, our system is disturbed with these anti-natural acts.

In the cosmic system, everything happens on time. The sun rises and sets on time. Seasons come on time and the flowers and fruits appear when there is time for them. I am writing this book during the monsoons of 2002. There are no monsoons in northwest India. I am in my home in the Himalayan Mountains and see the leaves on trees getting pale. I do not see all the birds, butterflies and other insects, which come during this time of the year. We human beings also cannot tolerate heat any more and many people are getting sick. There are no monsoons and the cosmic system is perturbed in this part of the world. Similarly, when our body functions are not performed properly, we also get unwell like the atmosphere appears now. What is interesting to note is that despite the drought, the usual herbs of the season are still growing but with a faded and droopy appearance as if they are going to die. Similarly, if we do not take care of ourselves and lead a life that is against the system of nature, we get a withered look.

Individual variations

People differ from one another because of a slight difference in their fundamental constitution called prakriti in Ayurveda. This difference is due to the variation in the proportion of the three main energies. This is what makes us different from one another and unlike machines, as the system of modern medicine tends to see us. Prakriti not only describes the variations in physiological features of individuals but also their personality types. The fundamental constitution of an individual is a very important theme of Ayurvedic treatment. For putting into practice the methods described in this book, you need to know your fundamental constitution or prakriti.

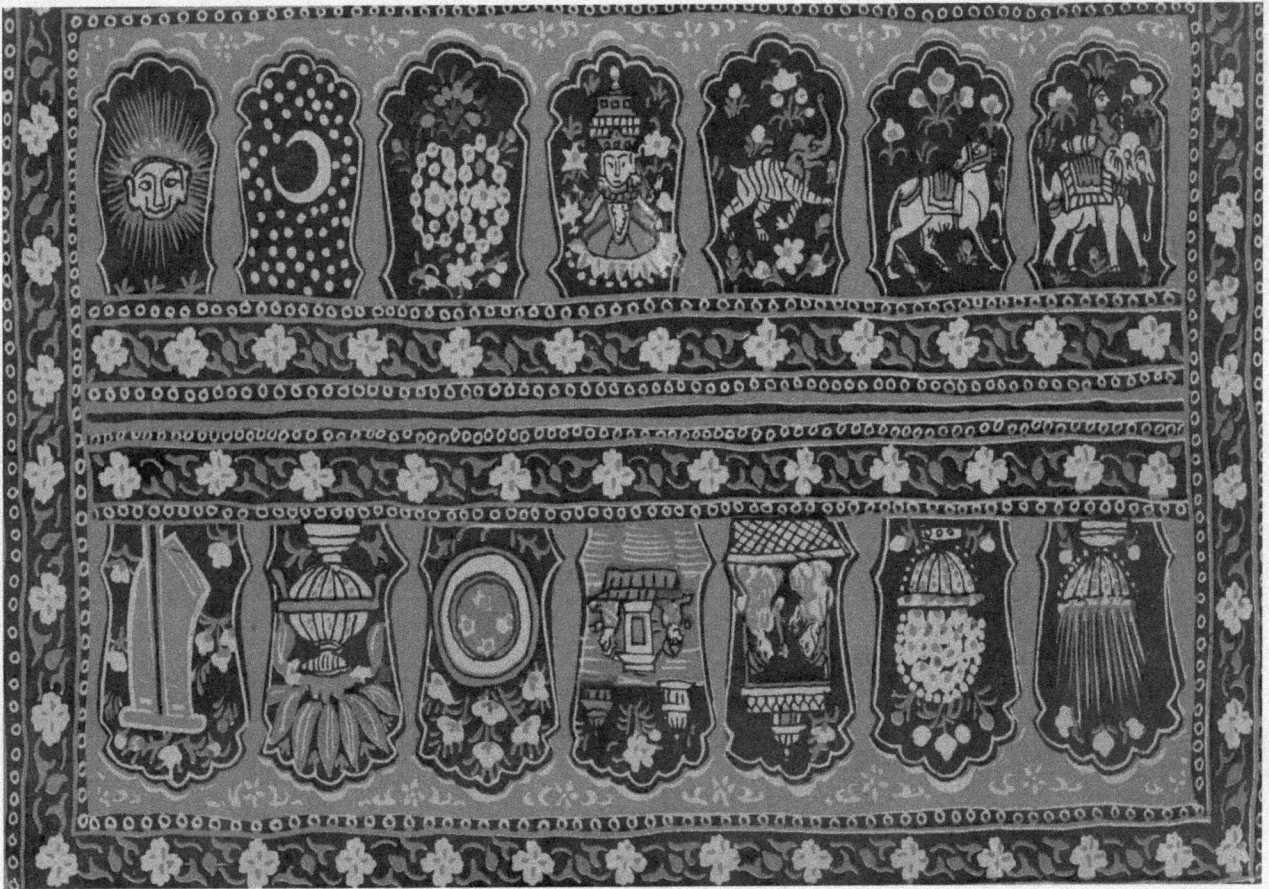

Prakriti

According to Ayurveda, each one of us has an individual constitution from birth. It is the basis of our physiological and psychological reactions. For maintaining good health, it is necessary to take the individual constitution into consideration.

The prakriti of an individual is due to the dominance of one or more energy and attributes the individual the characteristics of that particular dosha in slightly more predominance than the others. For example, the pitta prakriti individuals are sensitive to heat, sweat a lot and eat and drink in plenty. The vata prakriti ones are agile and swift in their movements. The kapha prakriti persons are slow and stable in their movements and are more tolerant than the previous two. In the mixed prakriti, the person may experience different attributes at different times and in different situations.

Seven types of prakriti

VATA	VATA-PITTA	SAMADOSHA (all energies in equal proportions)
PITTA	PITTA-KAPHA	
KAPHA	VATA-KAPHA	

Determining your prakriti

You need to know the characteristics of each type of prakriti in order to understand yourself.

Physical features and personality traits of individuals with vata prakriti

1.	Intolerant to cold and shiver easily
2.	Agile
3.	Quick and unrestricted in their movements
4.	Swift in actions
5.	Dry skin
6.	Smoky eyes and rather dull complexion
7.	Coarse hair and nails
8.	Prominent blood vessels
9.	Quick to worry, get easily fearful and in general rapid in the display of emotions
10.	Get easily irritated

Physical features and personality traits of individuals with pitta prakriti

1. Intolerant to heat
2. Have usually hot face
3. Delicate organs
4. Tendency to have moles, freckles and pimples
5. Lustrous complexion and reddish eyes
6. Excessive hunger and thirst
7. Tendency to have hair fall
8. Body odour
9. Intolerance and lack of endurance
10. Get easily angry specially when hungry

Physical features and personality traits of individuals with kapha prakriti

1. Slow in activities and speech
2. Stable movements
3. Well united and strong ligaments
4. Clear eyes, face and complexion
5. Little hunger, thirst or perspiration
6. Disorderly
7. Delayed initiation
8. Slow to take decisions
9. Patient and tolerant
10. Generally satisfied

I have given above the major features of three diverse kinds of prakriti. I am sure your thought process is rapidly trying to find 'Who am I?' Some of you may get confused to find out that you have characteristics of the two of the three energies described above. Obviously, you have mixed prakriti.

Mixed prakriti
As you know from the above description, you can be vata-pitta, vata-kapha and pitta- kapha. When you have mixed prakriti, different signs may appear in phases, in different situations or in different parts of the body. For example, you may be quick to react and decide, active in doing things and keeping order at times whereas at other times you may be slow, lazy and indecisive. During this latter period, you may be calm and take well thought out decisions whereas in your active period, you may take impulsive decisions for which you

may have to regret at times. Certain parts of your body may have smooth skin whereas other parts may have dry and rough skin. These features mean, you are of **vata-kapha** prakriti. Recall the elements of these two energies. You have predominance of wind and vastness of space on one side and stillness of earth and water on the other side. You have the dryness of wind and wetness of water. If you are of **vata-pitta** prakriti, at times you feel terribly intolerant to heat and at other times you feel intolerant to cold and want heat. You may have excessive sweating in some parts of the body whereas in other parts, you may have dryness. Your requirement to eat and drink may vary from time to time. Similarly, your complexion may vary from lustrous to dull. Thus, you have features of both vata and pitta. You have the fiery element, as well as wind. The wind makes the fire waver from low to high and takes away its stability. Similarly, fire produces heat and that brings the wind in movement.

If you have **pitta-kapha** prakriti, you have fire on the one hand and water on the other with completely contrasting characteristics. However, the heaviness of the earth brings stability in this contrasting state. Dynamic at times, you may postpone your work at another time. One day, you may wake up with great enthusiasm and dynamism to clear the disorder around you. Sometimes or during some phase of your life, you may eat a lot whereas at other times, have a relatively small appetite. You may be intolerant, impatient and quick to get angry at one time whereas at another time, you may surprise others with your tolerance and patience.

If you feel that you are a balanced person and your physical needs are stable, you have **samadosha** prakriti. Individuals with this prakriti are not disturbed by changing weather or climate, change of place and changing moods of others. They are mentally quite stable individuals.

For determining prakriti in a systematic manner, work out in three steps. Observe carefully your external appearance, then your physical reactions and then behaviour. I have summed up the process in the following table.

Your prakriti is your body's basic nature and the tendency of the nature is to be orderly and healthy. Due to external factors like weather, climate, stress, wrong nutrition, and so on, prakriti may change into vikriti or imbalance, which is a state of non-health[*]. Nature of the body is such that it reverts back to its natural conditions on its own. But if the factors disturbing this nature

---

[*] I have coined this word non-health to translate vikriti. Vikriti is not a state of ill health. It is a temporary diversion from the state of health, when the organisation of the body is disturbed.

are very strong and constantly oppress it, the state of vikriti is prolonged. We need appropriate food, drugs and other measures to revert back to prakriti. However, if the state of imbalance or the disorganised body conditions are left unattended for a long time, it will give rise to ailments or disorders.

Prakriti determination

External Appearance	Physical Reactions	Behaviour
The most basic observation for determining prakriti as well as to know the state of your health is your outward appearance. It includes observing eyes, complexion, nature of the skin, quantity and quality of the hair, body structure and other features of an individual.	The second step to determine prakriti is to observe your physical reactions to various life situations. For example to note the physical reactions to a stress situation, a shocking news, a good news, an exciting news, an emergency, and so on. When under stress or in a bad situation, some may have frequent stool or urination (pitta), the others may get constipation (vata), there are still others who may vomit (kapha). Some may just sleep or remain dumbfounded (kapha). On long-term stress situations like at work, various persons display diverse reactions. Some may get stomach problems or other ailments related to digestive system (pitta). There are others, who may get different kinds of aches (vata). Another type of persons may start sleeping too much and also get a little depressed (kapha).	The way people walk, talk, climb up the stairs, enter into a room, answer their doorbells or telephones reveal their prakriti. Vata prakriti individuals jump up the stairs, almost jump to respond to telephone or doorbell. In between are pitta and the slower ones are kapha. Notice the behavioural aspect of their reactions. When something goes wrong, people react differently. Does a person gets angry (pitta) or keeps patience (kapha)? While narrating something, various persons have their own ways. Similarly, while listening to others, people react differently. The ones full of enthusiasm and clarity in narration are of pitta prakriti. Those who are too rapid and confuse the story slightly are the individuals with vata prakriti. Slow and stable narration comes from kapha prakriti individuals.

Prakriti and vikriti (state of non-health)

It is normal to change from the state of prakriti to vikriti due to so many reasons in our day-to-day life. A normal healthy person automatically reverts back to prakriti. However, if you assist nature in her task, the process to revert back to prakriti will be rapid. Charaka, the great Ayurvedic sage of 6th Century B.C. had compared it to a person who falls after tripping on a stone. The person will get up any way; however, if someone gives him/her a hand, it is helpful.

Prakriti 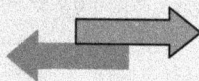 Vikriti

You can recognise vikriti by various symptoms. As I said earlier, these are mostly 'subjective symptoms'. Always remember that you are the best judge of your body. No machine and no physician can know your body better than you yourself. Thus do not ignore any signs and be always alert to the slight changes taking place in your body and state of mind.

Following table sums up the lists of symptoms caused by vikriti in your three energies. You may have one or more of these symptoms. It is not essential that you have all the symptoms simultaneously. The more acute the vikriti, the more intense are the symptoms. But your aim should be to nip the evil in the bud by reacting immediately to the slightest derangement from prakriti.

From the table given below, you will be able to find out when prakriti becomes vikriti. There are certain things that you may be already experiencing but may not necessarily think that they signify a diversion from your state of health. Some examples are hiccupping, yawning, sweet taste in mouth, undue anger and irritation, pimples or change in your complexion. Once you understand scientifically the entire system of Ayurveda, you will realise the interconnection between the nagging problems you have and the balance of three main energies of the body.

Symptoms of Dosha Vikriti

VATA	PITTA	KAPHA
• You get up in the morning with a stiff body. • You have often constipation or hard and dark coloured stool. Urine is grey or muddy. • Your skin is too dry despite the fact you often oil it. • You have dull and ashy complexion and smoky eyes. • You get very often a dried throat and feel like drinking even during the night. • You have restless sleep or have trouble sleeping. • You yawn often and tend to get hiccups. • You have fatigue that goes away after rest, sleep or hot bath. • You have a lack of tolerance and lack of endurance. • You feel often irritated and impatient.	• You perspire too much and have a body odour. • You get yellow to dark yellow urine and thin stool. • You get reddish eyes. • Your complexion looks reddish and you may get skin eruptions or pimples. • You have abnormal hunger and thirst. Excessive eating does not make you fat. • Often you may get minor stomach related problems. • You often get pimples, herpes or blisters or tearing of the skin. • You feel excessive heat in your body. • You feel dissatisfied. • You get often bouts of anger.	• You do not want to get up in the morning. You have a heavy feeling and wish to sleep the whole day. You feel drowsy during the day. • You get whiteness in urine, eyes and faeces. • You get whitish complexion without any glow and skin remains moist. • You have a sweet taste in your mouth. • You get excessive salivation. • You often get a cold sensation. • You get itchy feeling in your throat. • You get nausea from time to time. • You have a sense of lassitude. • You get inertness and also depression at times.

Imagine one morning, your stool is hard and dark. During the day you feel fatigued and yawn. If you catch these minor symptoms there and then, and do something, you will be fine by next day. However, if you ignore them, they will persist until the next morning and you will have slightly stiff body upon getting up and despite the night's rest, you will feel tired. This state will also affect your external appearance and you may find that you have a dull appearance. You will see that if you will take measures to treat vitiated vata, all the symptoms that make you feel unwell will disappear. However, if you do not take measures and let this state go on, it will spoil the internal environment of your body and you will get a dull appearance over a period of time. In the long run, you may get sleep disturbances, various aches and pains, blood related ailments, and so on. My principal purpose here is to make you conscious about your state of health and its relationship with your appearance and immediately find out the state of vikriti or non-health. Finding that you have diverted from state of health to non-health, you need to take measures to restore health without delay. Before you learn that, you need to learn few more things to comprehend the holistic system of Ayurveda and use it optimally to restore your health and glamour.

The biological aspect of vikriti

Vata, pitta and kapha are the three energies that are responsible for all the mental and physical functions of your body. They work in coordination with each other. For example, the function of vata is distribution of energy in the body. The formation of energy by digesting food is the function of pitta. For the digestion of food, we need digestive juices. Digestive juices are produced by kapha. They are carried from one place to another by vata. Once the energy is produced by pitta, vata distributes it to each and every part of the body. If the quality of the digestive juices is not good or pitta is sluggish to perform its functions or vata is too quick or too slow, the total system is disturbed. You can compare this to the postal system. You are waiting for a letter from a friend. You ask your postman everyday if there is a letter for you. He has none. A letter sent by post is a collaborative work of so many people at different destinations and postman can give you only what he is given to deliver. For a letter to reach its destination, everybody related to this task should perform his/her function properly. Similarly, if someone has cold hands and cold feet, the error can be at the level of the quantity of energy (pitta), faulty distribution (vata) or low quantity and quality of digestive juices (kapha).

Vikriti or the diversion from normal and natural is under or over function of one of the three energies, lack of coordination in the functions of the three energies or their displacement. The examples of under and over-functions of vata are low and high blood pressure. Under function of pitta is indigestion and heartburns or acidity denote displacement or over function. Excessive sleep and drowsiness is over function or displacement of kapha. Lack of secretions is an under-function of kapha.

Your dry skin is due to under function of kapha and over function of vata. Excessively oily skin is over function of kapha and pitta. Excessively moist skin is an over function of kapha. Under function of pitta will make you look pale whereas over function will give you reddish skin, pimples, skin irruptions, and so on. Excessive vata makes your skin rough and dry.

Interrelationship of body and mind

You have seen from the above description that the three energies of the body not only determine your physical appearance but also your personality traits. For example, pitta prakriti individuals are quick to get angry, especially before meal times; persons of kapha prakriti are rather indecisive and vata prakriti ones are rash and rather too quick to decide. Your thought process and mental state influence the three energies and similarly the imbalance of the three energies influences your thought process. With self-control, you can diminish or enhance the anger, irritation or inertness already present in your personality. If you enhance the anger, it also influences pitta and vitiates it in due course of time. If you control your anger, you can keep pitta in equilibrium. You should think that pitta is fire energy. An angry state of mind produces more uncontrolled fire. Uncontrolled fire is always dangerous and gives negative results.

The three dimensions of the mind

Like the three energies of the body, the mind has also three characteristic qualities or dimensions. These are:
- rajas,
- tamas
- sattva.

Along with the equilibrium of the three energies, it is essential to maintain equilibrium in the three dimensions of the mind. The rajas dimension of mind includes thinking, planning and taking decisions. The tamas dimension of mind hinders motion in contrast to rajas. Tamas also includes all what hinders the expansion of the mind (greed, anger, jealousy, laziness, etc.). The sattva dimension of the mind includes equilibrium, goodness, truth, compassion, stillness and peace.

Sattva- the mind balancer

Our everyday life is full of rajas and tamas. We need to work in order to earn our living (rajas). When we are exhausted from work, there is a moment of non-activity (tamas). Day is predominant with rajas whereas night is predominant with tamas. In everyday life, the negative aspects of tamas like greed, anger, jealousy, etc. are also present. Sattva helps to create a balance in mental activities and provides us stillness and peace. In practice, sattva is to maintain stillness and peace of mind in diverse situations in life. Sattva is that inner light which enlightens our way in life, gives us peaceful and restful sleep and helps maintain an equilibrium of the body and the mind. In fact, the sattva dimension of the mind creates equilibrium in rajas and tamas. In our modern life, there is a lack of sattva and excess of rajas and tamas. Lack of sattva enhances competition, jealousy, greed etc. and gives rise to frustration. Charaka lays a great emphasis on santosha (satisfaction) and sattva for maintaining good health. If you learn to attain a mental state of peace and satisfaction, it will not only keep you away from many modern day ailments, but also will enhance your charm. Look at yourself in the mirror when you are dissatisfied and frustrated. You acquire an unattractive look that you yourself dislike. Satisfaction is a state of mind that does not come with acquiring things or being rich. Sattvic mental state helps you to acquire a radiant look because it removes the cover of darkness from around the inner source of the cause of being– the soul and emits the pure energy.

An imbalance of sattva, rajas and tamas not only influences the equilibrium of the three energies but also causes mental ailments. Thus, for maintaining good health and longevity, a six dimensional equilibrium is essential as the three dimensions at two levels mutually influence each other. Any imbalance of the three qualities of mind also influences the equilibrium of humours and vice versa.

The six dimensions of human existence along with the soul– the driving force of our being.

A state of vikriti also influences the mind. If constipation or partial evacuation persists, it can give rise to sleep disorders or a disturbed mental state or nervous behaviour. Stomach problems, which are due to pitta disturbances, may enhance anger and irritation.

One cannot think of doing everything relating to the three doshas and expect to be in perfect health. Equally important is to maintain a mental level of equilibrium with a state of stillness, calm and satisfaction. It is sattva that maintains the balance between activities (rajas) and non-activities (tamas).

A Complete Human Being of Ayurveda

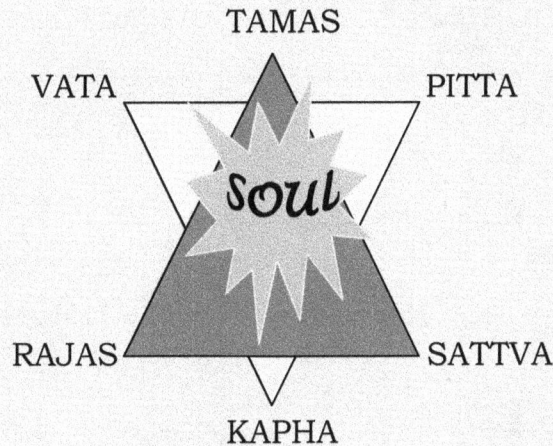

Influence of external factors on your body and mind

In Ayurveda, we are told to live according to desha (space) and kala (time). Internal and external forces are constantly affecting your prakriti. You have to learn to create a balance and to counteract those forces which adversely affect your equilibrium. Windy and stormy weather can cause imbalance of vata. If we take measures like massage, fomentation, specific nutritional supplements like ginger, garlic, fenugreek, ajwain and other vata reducing products, the effect of windy weather will be counterbalanced. Similarly, excess of heat can cause an imbalance of pitta. Cold baths, cooling ointments like sandalwood paste, yellow earth (multani mitti), cool rooms and nutrients containing sweet, bitter and astringent tastes can reduce the effect of heat on us and save us from pitta imbalance. Humid and cold weather tends to vitiate kapha. A vapour bath or hot bath, sour and spicy meals and some exercise will counteract the effect of the weather and prevent any kapha vitiation. Think in terms of the element that dominates you and the element that dominates at that particular time in the atmosphere. If however, you take the contrary actions to the above-said, obviously, you will have imbalance of your already dominating energy. For example if you are kapha dominating and cold and wet weather has its effect and makes you lazy. Instead of eating hot and spicy food, you eat fatty and sweet food. That will further disturb your kapha and will make you sleep long and feel drowsy during the day. You may get some other symptoms of kapha disturbance as well. However, if you get used to bringing minor alterations in your lifestyle according to the change of weather, your body's energies will simultaneously coordinate with the cosmic energies.

Effect of the time of the day, age and climate at a particular geographical location on dosha

ENERGY	TIME	AGE	CLIMATE
KAPHA	Morning Evening	Childhood	Humid, cold
PITTA	Noon Midnight	Youth	Dry, hot
VATA	Afternoon Late Night	Middle age and old age	Dry, cold, windy

Note: The hot and humid climate is pitta-kapha promoting.

Methods and remedies to revert back to prakriti from vikriti

You should know in a comprehensive manner what steps to take when you diagnose that you have diverted from prakriti to vikriti. You can make a multidimensional effort to revert back to prakriti and thus, help nature to maintain its order and bless you with well-being and beauty. Multidimensional efforts like nutrition, yoga, herbal remedies, sattvic thoughts, appropriate rest, etc., will enable you to re-establish your harmony and regain your usual strength and vitality rapidly.

Remedies for vata vikriti: Symptoms of vata vikriti are: Dry skin, dull complexion, dry throat, stiff body, constipation, disturbed sleep and nervousness. It is important to look into the factors that cause vata imbalance in your particular case, especially if it happens often. Some persons may get this disturbance due to certain foods like some kind of lentils or beans, over-ripe peas or a certain kind of bread with yeast. It is extremely important to eradicate these factors that divert your prakriti to vikriti. Take the following measures to treat vata vikriti:

- Drinking hot water is a remedial measure for vata vitiation.
- Do the oil saturation massage with warm oil (see Chapter 4).
- Take warm bath, dry fomentation and appropriate rest.
- Eat warm and unctuous food predominant in sweet and sour rasas. Avoid pungent, astringent and bitter substances.
- Take only hot foods and drinks and avoid all cold foods and drinks.
- Recommended foods are milk, banana, papaya, citrus fruits, carrots, turnips, fenugreek (methi), kalonji, cumin, fennel, dill seeds, cardamom and ginger.
- Take herbal tea with basil and liquorice. Add 4-5 basil leaves and a half-teaspoon of powdered liquorice in half litre water. Bring it to boil and let it cook for about five minutes on a low fire with the lid on. Put off the fire and let it stay like this for a few minutes.
- If your vata vitiation is caused due to an exposure to cold and you have stiffness and body ache, boil 6-7 crushed cardamoms and 7-8 leaves of basil in half litre water for five minutes. Keep the preparation covered and cook on a low fire. Drink it in two doses.
- If you are suffering from fatigue due to vata, take tea with big cardamom, clove and cinnamon. Crush one big cardamom, three cloves and a small piece of cinnamon and boil these in half a litre water. Let it cook covered on low fire for about five minutes. You may add some candy sugar into it to sweeten. This preparation can also be taken as normal tea or chai with the addition of black tea and milk.
- Ajwain or thyme tea is also good to alleviate vata vitiation. Dose for ajwain or thyme is half a teaspoon in half a litre of water. Make the tea as described above.
- Ginger, basil and cardamom tea is very effective in vitiated vata. Crush about 3 cubic centimetres of ginger, 5 basil leaves and 3 cardamoms. Add all this in half a litre of water and make the tea in a similar manner as has been described above. In case you do not have fresh ginger, replace it with half teaspoon of powdered ginger. Add some candy sugar in the end to make the spicy taste of the ginger milder.

- For treating vata imbalance, take one clove of garlic daily, crush it and add ¼ of a teaspoon of ghee and swallow. Do not drink anything cold after taking this preparation.
- Crush one teaspoon each of kalonji and cumin along with two teaspoons of candy sugar. Split this into six doses and take three times a day for two days. If you think that you are still not completely cured from the symptoms of vata vitiation, repeat this for another few days.
- If your vata vitiation is too frequent and intense, you should take the treatment for 15 days or more with chaturbeej churan (powder of four seeds). Powder the following four different kinds of seeds in equal quantity: fenugreek, ajwain, cress and kalonji. Take half a teaspoon of this powder 3 to 4 times a day.

Remedies for pitta vikriti: Symptoms of disturbed pitta are: excessive heat in your body, skin ruptures, herpes or pimples on your skin or you have indigestion, sour taste in your mouth, too much hunger or thirst or too much sweat, have yellow coloured urine and have a body odour or you may be quick to angry. One or more of these symptoms indicate that you have an imbalance of this energy.

Avoid all those factors that vitiate pitta. Do not take alcoholic beverages; eat simple food which is mildly spiced and salted. Avoid chillies, pepper or anything else that gives a burning sensation. Avoid being in the sun and the afternoon heat. Eradicate all those factors that bring more heat to your body. Take the following measures to bring the vitiated pitta to equilibrium:

- Drink plenty of water, cold milk and cooling sherbets like brahmi or sandalwood.
- Take a cold bath and apply cooling ointments like sandalwood paste, ghee or coconut oil on your body. If you have burning sensation in a specific part of the body, you may apply sandalwood paste only on that specific part of the body.
- Anoint yourself with mud. Yellow and fine variety of earth is used for this purpose. It is also called 'healing earth' or 'Multani mitti' in India. Make a thin paste with this earth by adding water and apply it to your body. Leave it for about half an hour and wash it off. This treatment will also make your skin smooth and shiny.
- Take foods that are dominant in sweet, bitter and astringent rasas. Suggested foods are rice, masoor dal, spinach, carrots, cabbage, pumpkin, courgette, aubergine, bitter gourd, dates, bananas, sweet

apples and grapes, papaya, cold milk, ghee, fresh cheese (paneer), fennel, clove, coriander and liquorice.

- Take herbal teas like wormwood, neem, coriander and liquorice. Take extremely bitter substances only in a very moderate quantity. Use a few leaves of neem or wormwood and mix them with some ajwain to make the tea. The reason for this is that exclusively bitter rasa may cure your vitiated pitta but in turn may vitiate your vata.
- Take a teaspoon of juice of bitter gourd two times a day to pacify the excessive heat in the body.
- Masoor dal soup with ghee is an effective dietary measure to cure vitiated pitta. The recipe is given below.

Masoor dal (red lentil) soup

Masoor dal	100gm or ½ cup
Fennel	¼ teaspoon
Curcuma	¼ teaspoon
Salt	to taste
Ghee	3 teaspoons
Coriander leaves (chopped)	1 tablespoon*

Clean and wash the dal a few times and let it soak for about 15 minutes. Boil ½ litre (2 ½ cups) of water and put the dal into it after draining out the water. Add spices and salt and cook on a low fire with a lid on for about half an hour. Stir from time to time. At the end if the preparation is thick, add more water to make it soupy and boil it after adding water. Add the chopped coriander leaves in the end and add ghee before serving.

If coriander leaves are not available, add crushed coriander seeds along with other spices.

Remedies for kapha vikriti: The symptoms of kapha vikriti are: a sweet taste in mouth, too much salivation, foamy urine, sticky stool and desire to sleep a lot. You may get a feeling of heaviness in your body and may feel drowsy, lazy and passive.

It is important to avoid all those factors that lead to kapha vitiation. Oily, fatty, salty and heavy to digest foods should be avoided. Sedentary habits and lack of exercise vitiate this energy further and therefore you should force yourself to be active and go out for a walk or undertake other activities.

To reverse the state of kapha vikriti into your natural state or prakriti, take the following measures:

- Use spices like ginger, garlic, dill seeds, kalonji, fenugreek and mustard seeds.
- Always have freshly prepared hot food.
- Hot bath and vapour bath are very effective in curing kapha vikriti.
- Force yourself to do physical exercise and go for walks.
- Make an effort to keep awake (less sleep).
- Make an effort to go out, meet people rather than sitting alone and feeling drowsy.
- Avoid watching too much television.
- Suggested foods are Soybeans, potatoes, cress salad, tomatoes, cauliflower, peaches, plumbs, citrus fruits and honey. Ghee should be avoided and cooking should be done in moderate quantity of sesame or olive oil. Sugar and products containing sugar should not be taken. To sweeten tea or coffee, use candy sugar.
- Take a clove of garlic everyday with some honey.
- Take herbal tea with ginger, cardamom, pepper and basil.

Summary of living an Ayurvedic way of life for health and beauty

For living the Ayurvedic way, follow systematically the steps given below:

- First of all, you need to know your prakriti. You cannot take care of yourself until you do not know your body's nature and mind's fundamental qualities.
- Always observe yourself well and moment you have vikriti, take measures to help nature to restore your state of health back to normal.
- Follow the Ayurvedic principles of nutrition regarding the quantity and quality of the food.
- Do not ignore weather, change of climate or change of place.
- Do not ignore your fatigue.
- Keep the body and mind clean
- Take rasayana (health promoting products) regularly and never forget to do some exercise.
- Give always an antidote to the nature of work you do.
- Imbibe sattva in your life and overcome fear.
- Avoid using chemical or other strong medicines. Keep patience and trust in helping nature to heal on its own.

2
Body: a Journey from Inner to Outer

The purpose of this chapter is to make you understand the influence of our body's internal environment and our inner subtle being on our outward appearance.. There are two aspects of the inner reality– organic and subtle. Various systems of the body and their functions work at organic level and form a part of our inner environment. The mental and spiritual aspect of our being is the subtle part of our inner environment. Our being is interconnected to the rest of the cosmos and at the same time, we are a continuity of our past through our past karma. For our health and outward appearance, we need to understand all this and take into account various aspects of our being.

The Inner Environment of the Body (organic)

The inner environment of the body at the organic level influences your strength and appearance. It is equally important to keep your internal parts clean as the external in order to be healthy and attractive. Deposits of dirt (mala) on internal parts of the body ruin the inner environment and make the functions of internal organs sluggish. They are the source of toxicity in the blood, thus giving rise to bad skin with pimples and rash, as well as allergies.

Factors that ruin the inner environment of the body and deposit mala

- **Constipation or partial evacuation:** Constipation or partial evacuation ruin the internal environment due to decay and spreading stink inside the body. Over a period of time, partial evacuation leads to the deposits of toxins in the blood stream that leads to various skin ailments and allergies. It weakens the immune system and one may get frequent attacks of common cold and other minor ailments. Thus, for maintaining good skin and complexion, make sure that you accustom your body to go to the toilette twice a day and have proper evacuation. Constipation or other difficulties related to evacuation are due to vata imbalance. If not attended to immediately, the vata imbalance enhances and gives rise to a series of vata related problems. Rough skin and dull complexion are also amongst those.

- **Mala in urine:** It is essential to maintain proper water-balance in the body so that urine throws out toxins regularly. Low water level leads to impure blood because the kidneys do not function properly and urine with toxins stays too long in the bladder, thus causing toxicity in the body. Drinking too much water and urinating too frequently is not the solution to this problem, as that over-strains the whole water system of the body. The right way to maintain water balance is to drink warm water (preferably cardamom water as described below) in the morning upon getting up, before each meal and shortly before retiring for the night. Your meals should be warm and fluid (soups, various vegetables and fruits and meats with sauce). Rice and pasta contain large amount of water. Make sure that your urine is transparent and not yellow or turbid.

- **Deposits of other malas:** Your body throws out mala in several other forms. If skin, nose ears, eyes and mouth are not cleaned properly, the mala deposits in these parts and ruins the inner environment of the body. For example, if the nasal passage is not cleaned properly, the passage of the prana energy or the life giving force that we breathe in is constantly hindered. That can give rise to pale complexion and headache or other ailments related to sense organs. The same is true of washing off sweat and other skin excretions with daily bath, care and cleaning of buccal cavity (mouth and tongue), ears and eyes[*].

- **Eating too much, too frequently and heavy to digest nutrients:** Eating too much leads to fat deposits and makes the liver sluggish. Needless to say that excessive fat makes you over-weight, ruins the form of your body, have grievous effects on your heart and blood circulation and opens way for several other ailments.[**] A sluggish liver gives you a pale complexion. Eating too frequently and before the first meal is digested, leads gradually to amadosha. Amadosha is a condition when partially digested food remains and hinders the digestive process. If amadosha is not treated, it gradually transfers the malas and toxins in the main blood stream, thus leading to various allergies and skin problems. Hard to digest nutrients, if taken frequently also tax your digestive system causing ill health, bad complexion and deteriorate the skin quality.

---

[*] For more details on this theme, consult my book: *Ayurveda a Way of Life*. Latest edition is available at www.amazon.com and at Pilgrims Book House in Delhi, Varanasi and Kathmandu.
[**] Refer to my book: *Losing Weight with Yoga and Ayurveda*, available at www.amazon.com

- **Interfering in the natural cleansing process of the body:** If we happen to eat something that does not suit us or is contaminated or toxic, the body reacts in a natural way and throws out these toxins. You may get diarrhoea, vomiting, fever and excessive sweat. These are nature's ways of getting rid of what acts on your body as anti-life. If you interfere in this process and take medication to stop this cleansing process, you are going against nature and letting your body accumulate toxins.

- **Phlegm deposits in nasal, bronchial or sinus cavities:** Blockage of nasal passage should be avoided because this hinders the flow of prana energy into your body and causes migraines, vision problems and damages the other senses. If remains unattended for a long time, it gives rise to deterioration in memory and retention and may lead to partial paralysis. Phlegm deposit in sinus cavities in the skull cause serious health problems and give you a sickly appearance.

- **Hindering the natural urges:** Charaka has described that there are certain urges of the body that should not be hinderedbecause it leads to ill health. Urge to stool, urinate, yawn, hiccup, tears, semen, breathing fast after physical strain, and so on should not be suppressed. They lead to various ailments and make you feel dull and drab.

- **Hindered flow of milk in case of nursing mothers:** due to some psychological factors like fear, nervousness, etc. the flow of milk is hindered in some cases after delivery. The mammary glands are prepared for secretion of the milk and if due to an unhealthy life-style or above mentioned reasons the flow of milk is hindered, it gives rise to various health complications and may have long term negative effects on your health and appearance.

Ways to safeguard the inner environment of the body

- To ensure proper evacuation, drink hot water boiled with cardamom after getting up in the morning. Cardamom has properties to balance the three doshas and it energises and perfumes the water. You need to add 2 to 3 cardamoms for 1 to 1 ½ litre of water and boil the water for a minute. You can make this preparation for two three days and heat the water before drinking. Drink one big glass of water. If you are suffering from constipation or partial evacuation, drink two glasses of water. Do not lie down after drinking water. Walk or do some exercises or yoga. I suggest that you tune your system for evacuating twice a day. Include lot of fruits and salads in your diet. Papaya is highly recommended. Drink hot water as described above, one hour before dinner and make an effort to evacuate. Even if you are not able to, keep going to the toilet ritualistically and apply little pressure. Ultimately, your system will get tuned to it.

- Daily cleansing of the nasal passage should be done by blowing nose with force immediately after a hot shower or bath. From time to time, you should apply some mustard oil in the nasal passage and try to sneeze. This should also be done after your shower when phlegm is slightly softened due to heat. Yogic jalaneti or cleansing of nasal passage with water is another very effective method to keep the nasal passage clean and obstruction free*.
- Daily bath or shower with warm water is highly recommended in Ayurveda. Bath with coldwater twice a day is recommended in case of excessive heat. Take bath properly by rubbing the skin and using a massage brush. This process will clean the skin pores, activate the skin and make you look good. Anointing of the body with oil after bath will be described later.
- Some principles of Ayurvedic nutrition to make your inner climate agreeable and make you feel and look good will be given later in the chapter on nutrition.
- If you feel sick and think that it is due to some food or drink you have taken, immediately drink hot water and try to throw the half ingested food out. Do not let it continue to further spoil your inner environment. If you get vomiting and diarrhoea due to some contaminated food or other substances, let nature take its course of cleansing and do not hinder the process by taking drugs to cure yourself.

Methods of inner cleaning or Panchakarma

Ayurveda recommends inner cleaning of the body every six months after the two major seasons. The time recommended is September-October and March-April. The purpose of the inner cleaning is to throw out the toxins from the body and create equilibrium of the three energies of the body or doshas. These practices cleanse your inner organs and rejuvenate them. This cleaning process lends you a glow and gives you a smooth skin.

The classical Panchakarma has five internal cleaning practices but through my experience and research, I have realised that in our times we regularly need to do blood purification (detoxification) as well as the purification of our urinary system. Therefore I have made Panchakarma into Saptakarma or seven cleaning practices. I have also modified some of the practices so that you are

* See my book, *Programming your Life with Ayurveda* for details of Jalaneti

36

able to do them on your own without the help of an Ayurvedic physician. They are described at length in my various books on Ayurveda. Refer to *Programming your Life with Ayurveda* for doing Saptakarma on your own. I cite below the table of Saptakarma from this book in order to give you a general idea about the inner cleaning practices.

A summary of the complete Saptakarma

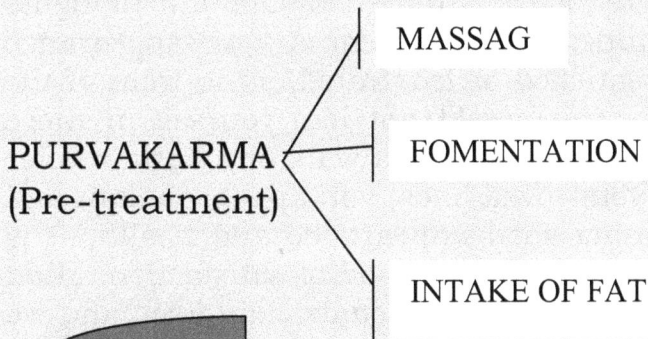

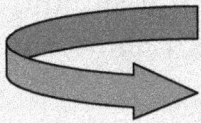

PURVAKARMA
(Pre-treatment)

MASSAG

FOMENTATION

INTAKE OF FAT

SAPTAKARMA (Seven cleansing practices)
1. Vamana or emesis (voluntary vomiting)
2. Virechana (purgation)
3. Anuvasana Basti (unctuous enema)
4. Asthapana Basti (non-unctuous enema)
5. Nasya (purification of the head region)
6. Raktashodhana (blood purification)
7. Bastishodhana (diuresis)

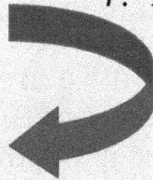

PASHCHATKARMA
(After-care)
1. Light, warm and liquid food
2. Intake of fluids
3. Rest and sleep
4. No hectic activity for two days

From the above practices, I will suggest diverse massages, fomentation and fat treatment which are a part of purvakarma. They are done to pacify vata. From the principal practices, you need to attain the knowledge of enemas. Enemas are important to uproot vata imbalance. Vata is responsible for skin and blood circulation and its imbalance make your appearance unattractive. In our modern times, due to hectic pace of life, too many activities and preserved foods, most people suffer from vata imbalance from one way or the other.

Purgation and blood purification are also used in some cases to attain a good and smooth skin. In the next chapter, wherever there is a reference to these practices, I will describe them in detail.

Inner environment at a subtle level

Our way of thinking and our deeds form the inner environment at a profound and subtle level. Inside the physical body, is the subtle body and our thoughts have a direct effect on it. The subtle body influences our appearance immediately. When you feel angry, dissatisfied or frustrated, sit in front of the mirror and watch your face. Certainly you would not like yourself in these moments. On the contrary, when you feel happy after a walk or a bath or after hearing a good news or upon meeting your loved ones, you appear radiant and get a glow on your face. For maintaining good appearance and health, it is essential to have a peaceful mental state and an attitude of satisfaction. Mind is a wanderer by nature but it has the capabilities of controlling itself and we should utilise this capacity of the mind. It can be developed with some simple techniques.

The limitless mind

In the great Indian epic *The Mahabharata*, one of the questions of Yaksha to Yudhishthra was– 'What is the fastest thing in the world.' 'Mind' was the response. Besides being fast, our thinking process is beyond space and time. It can diversify from geographically far away places to what was thousands of years ago and what is going to be in unseen future. We can heal ourselves and enhance our charm with the power of mind if we are able to focus its energy by stopping its constant diversification. The power of the mind I s evoked by controlling the thought process and harnessing the internal energy. On the contrary, losing control of one's thought process becomes the cause of many ailments and ultimately mental disorders. In the Katho Upanishad (III, 3), human beings and their existence in this world are compared to a journey in a chariot. The soul is the owner of the chariot, the intellect or buddhi is its driver and mind plays a part of reins whereas the senses are the horses. The world is the arena for this journey of the chariot. If the reins are not in control, the chariot can go off the road, and can break down. The buddhi should be used to control the reins of the mind in order to have a smooth journey of life. The horses (senses) should be taken care of in order to avoid any hindrance in the journey and for the well being of the entire chariot and its owner.

Without indulging in too many theoretical details, I cite below a case study for conveying the practical applications of my ideas.

I had a group of students from Switzerland and France in our Himalayan Centre. One morning, Isabelle (name changed) woke up with a terrible pain and twisted neck. She could not straighten her neck any more. Rational therapy gave her some relief but I knew that the cause was deeper than just a wrong posture during sleep. The students had an afternoon free a day earlier and they told me that they witnessed a funeral of a woman across the river and some of them filmed it also. On cross-questioning, it turned out that Isabelle's neck was stiffened in the same posture as she was watching the funeral. While she was watching the funeral, she was greatly moved by it as she relived the death of her mother that happened a few years ago. It is interesting that the previous evening at dinnertime, Isabelle was in a good shape and all the students were very enthusiastically telling me about the funeral pyre. The deceased was a middle aged woman and they dressed her body in new clothes and jewellery before putting her on the logs of wood for burning. Isabelle's internal suffering appeared in the form of torture to her body. It was her mother's demise and perhaps the fear of her own death that stirred her tremendously.

Influence of mind on your appearance

Two thousand six hundred years ago, Sushruta very aptly said that for good health and healing it is absolutely essential to remain 'prasanna chitta' or in a contented and happy state of mind. All of us are aware that when we feel happy and satisfied, we look good. Perhaps many people are not aware that when we remain in an unhappy state of mind or are depressed due to some reason or are in aggressive and grumpy state of mind, even our hair shows that. People often go on shampooing their hair blaming the falling and lifeless condition of their hair on water or shampoo or other superficial factors.

Happiness and satisfaction are not dependent upon wealth, possessions and status, etc. It is the mind that makes people happy or unhappy. The fundamental causes of unhappiness or dissatisfaction are greed, excessive desires, possessiveness, etc. Thus, it is more of a personal effort to assimilate the wisdom and learn to keep happy. What is most important is that you become aware of the fact that it is important for you to remain contented in all circumstances. You must realise that you are doing this for yourself, for your health and for your attractive appearance. Forget about the good karma or the next life or hell or heaven. Think of the most precious moment of your life, that is NOW and you are losing it by grumbling and complaining.

I suggest that in bad circumstances, you always keep in mind the ideas like–'I was saved', 'things could have been worse', 'there are more unhappy people around me than I am' and so on. Check yourself immediately if you are grumbling or grumpy. Be always grateful to nature for another day of life. Try to make each day of your life beautiful and happy. *Carpe diem* (seize the day) is a Latin adage that advises us to live tenderly and joyfully each moment of life. It is unnecessary to worry over what is already past and it is foolish to be afraid of a situation not yet come. Your state of mind reflects on your appearance. If you keep happy and satisfied, you laugh and smile in a natural manner, you would look radiant. There are people who are not contented and they remain perpetually frustrated. They smile in a measured manner and laugh rarely. They look withered even when they have good features and complexion.

Influence of mind on the three energies

I have described in the last chapter that for good health and attractive looks, we require a six dimensional equilibrium. It is important for you to know how our mind disturbs our state of health and precisely which energy and why.

Vata and your mind: In the above example of Isabelle, her profound emotions disturbed her vata. She lost the mobility of her neck and had pain. At another level, a worried or fearful state of mind may give rise to sleep disturbance or constipation or both. These factors effect nerves and disturb your sleep, make your behaviour nervous and you acquire a dull and withered complexion. On the contrary, if you are able to keep an emotional balance even in difficult situations through the strength and power of your mind, you can safeguard the balance of vata energy.

Pitta and your mind: If you remain dissatisfied, grumble often and have outburst of anger, it affects your pitta energy. Such people are prone to frequent problems with their digestive system. They suffer from acidity and heart burn. This suffering leads to further dissatisfaction and you get into a vicious cycle. Your skin and complexion will look reddish and uneven. At times you may also look very pale due to under-function of pitta energy. You may also get pimples, skin eruptions or dark patches on your skin.

Kapha and your mind: If you are often very passive in your thinking and spend lot of time in an indecisive state of mind, you will gradually disturb your kapha energy. You would rather sleep than take a decision. Sleeping excessively will make you more passive and you will tend to postpone your work. There will be a kind of confusion in your life, which may lead to depression. All this will disturb the kapha energy further. This gives rise to a lazy and drowsy appearance and a lifeless complexion. The excessive salivation and itchy feeling in the throat are other unpleasant factors that give you an unpleasant feeling.

By directing your mind towards a state of activity and wakefulness and maintaining discipline in your life, you can save yourself from kapha vikriti.

In brief, our mind influences our three principal energies and these in turn influence our health, as well as our appearance in a positive or negative way. At a physiological level, when our inner environment is disturbed, the same happens. Let us see precisely the negative effects on our health and appearance when one of the energies is diverted from prakriti to vikriti.

Influence of imbalance of the three energies on our appearance

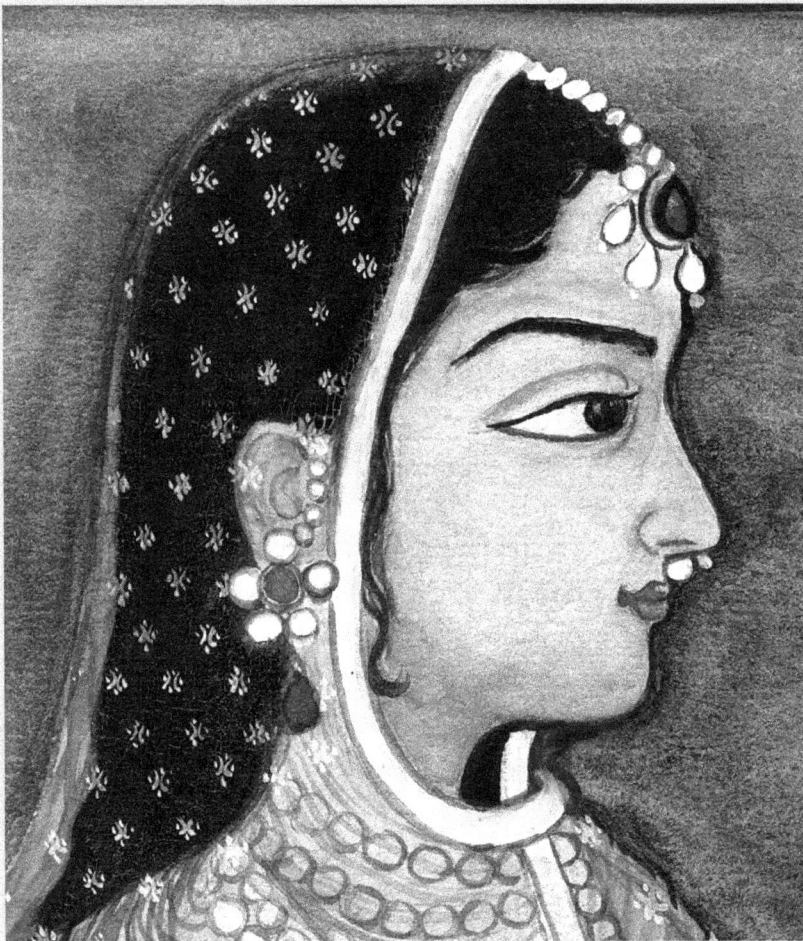

I have summarised below the direct influence of vikriti on your health and appearance. With the help of the table given below, you pin point your symptoms and take some measures described in the previous chapter to revert back to prakriti. The more you delay, the longer it will take you to get back to harmony and balance of three energies. If one of the disturbed energies is left unattended, in due course of time it will disturb the other two energies as they all work together to maintain the whole system. At this stage, you may become afflicted by an ailment.

Thus, for your health and attractive appearance, do something immediately to pacify the disturbed system.

Influence of vikriti on our appearance

Vata	Pitta	Kapha
• Dry and rough skin and ashy complexion • Coarse nails and hair • Nails break often and hairs have split ends • Slow down of hair growth • Slow down of growth in general in case of children • Dull complexion • Prominent blood vessels to give an appearance of older than one's age	• Reddish complexion • Skin with moles, freckles or pimples • Thickening and tearing of skin • Rash, acne and herpes. • Hair fall and danger of getting bald • Excessive perspiration and smell in the body • Burning sensation and itch to scratch	• Colourless and whitish complexion with lifeless appearance • Moist skin that gives rise to fungus in some areas of body like underarms, loins and feet • Itchy feeling in the throat and has to clear the throat often while speaking • Deformity of body organs and excessive growth

Controlling the mind

In Vedic tradition, the mind is considered as the sixth senses and superior to all senses because it controls the other senses. The mind itself should be harnessed by buddhi or the discerning ability of the mind that we human beings are blessed with. You should train yourself to use your buddhi. If I buy a computer and do not use it, it is not going to help me write a book. Similarly, many people buy equipment to trim themselves after they watch their impressive television advertisement but practically never use them. Thus, they remain over-weight as they were. Similarly, we all have the possibility to use our sense of discretion and we should make our maximum effort to do so. Given below are some practical suggestions to control the mind in three steps.

Three steps to control the mind

Proceed systematically to learn the methods of controlling your mind. Learn to control your senses and activities as the first step. The second step is the regulation of your breathing. The third step is nabhi ekagrata or concentration on your navel chakra.

Step I
Controlling the senses

Moderate use of senses: Excessive use of senses affects your appearance and gives you a worn out look. You will begin to look old and will suffer from excessive fatigue even at young age. It is important that you exercise mental control to avoid excessive use of your senses.

Speech and hearing: These are vata activities and excessive and continuous indulgence leads to vata imbalance.

- Do not indulge in worthless conversation. Avoid describing your life happenings and mundane events to people.
- Do not describe often and to too many people some bad happenings of your life. Whenever you describe such incidents, try to detach your self by being grateful that it is over.
- Try and get into the habit of exercising restraint on your speech. Use effective words to enhance your communication skills. Listen to yourself with involvement and analytical thoughts in order to improve and limit your conversation.
- Avoid noisy environment. If you have to work in conditions where you have to talk and listen, give yourself a quiet hour after work each day and try to have relatively quieter weekends in order to rebuild your energy.

Sense of smell: According to Ayurveda, the nose is also a passage to brain. Avoid buying products with synthetic perfumes. Excessive exposure to unpleasant smells disturbs the mind whereas an exposure to natural perfumes like jasmine, rose, sandalwood, etc. helps calm the mind.

- Take deep breaths by smelling some natural perfumes from flowers or extracts of other natural substances.
- Inhale vapours with etheric oils once a week. These will clear the nasal passage and throat, as well as will soothe your nerves.

Vision: Vision is the function of pitta. If you have to work long hours on computer, always use remedial measures to create an equilibrium. Use regularly some mild eye drops or wash your eyes with camille, basil or liquorice decoction from time to time.

- Do not ever read in a moving vehicle if the ride is bumpy.
- Wash your eyes upon getting up in the morning by splashing water with force on the open eyes.

Movements: If your movements are too little or are restricted to small spaces, you are likely to get kapha imbalance. However, excessive movements like too much travelling or walking leads to vata imbalance. If you have to travel a lot because of your work, compensate it with peaceful and calm holiday period. Try your best not to limit yourself to confined spaces. Many housewives and others who have their work place at home or near home tend to do that. Many of these people put on weight or get kapha imbalance. Going for a walk at some distance gives you the element ether which is essential for health and well being. Restraining yourself to smaller spaces gives a pale and lifeless complexion.

Step II
Rhythmical breathing

Learn to breathe properly: Breathing is not considered merely the intake of air for survival in both yoga and Ayurveda. We inhale the cosmic energy, called prana with each breath. The quality of this cosmic energy depends upon our environment. In the mountains and forest, inhalation is rejuvenating whereas in big cities with noise and air pollution, the prana energy is vitiated.

Do the following to get used to proper and rhythmical breathing:

- Take five deep breaths three times a day in the following manner. Do that upon getting up, before lunch and before going to bed. Inhale gradually to your full capacity, make a brief pause while holding the air inside. Exhale gradually and again give a very brief pause after all the air is out.
- After having done this for a month or so, use these breathing exercises to combat any stress situation and develop a peaceful mental state.

- Once you feel that you have mastered the conscious and rhythmical breathing, concentrate on your navel and breath five times like this thrice a day. This is preparatory for the next step for mental concentration.

Step III
Nabhi Ekagrata

Nabhi is navel and ekagrata is concentration on one particular point. This chakra or the concentric energy point is for the knowledge and well being of the body (Yogasutras of Patanjali, III, 29). Persistent concentration on the navel point will provide you not only a radiant look but also will make you aware of any imbalance in the body. A regular practice, twice a day for a few minutes is essential to achieve the goal. I will give below the easy method to learn this practice.

- **First week:** Do deep breathing as described above but send your breath to your navel. Hold it there before exhaling in a rhythmical manner. Do this practice for 2-3 minutes upon getting up and before going to bed.

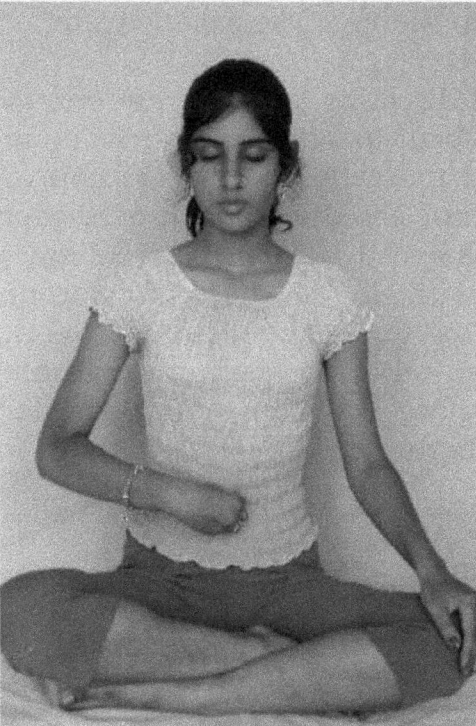

- **Second week:** Do the same as above but try to prolong the timings of inhalation, holding the breath, exhalation and pause after that.
- **Third week:** Put all the fingers of your right hand together and put them on your navel. Do the above-described breathing practice 11 times, twice a day. Your entire concentration should be on your navel and each time when you finish the breath, imagine the next number also on your navel.

- **Fourth week:** Do the practice 11 times with right hand fingers on your navel and another 11 times with the left hand fingers on your navel. This is the final version of this practice and I suggest that you make it a way of life. Do it twice daily.

Sattva for health and beauty

Sattva is a balancing energy of our daily activities. It is attained by stillness and purity of mind. Make an effort to get rid of the feelings of jealousy, anger, possessiveness, greed, etc. Try not to be a slave to your senses and use the reins of your mind to control them and divert them to a better cause. Develop an attitude of 'forget and forgive' and direct your thoughts for a constructive cause. Do not let your thinking process entertain thoughts which lead to destruction. Destructive thoughts about others make the mind restless and give rise to tamas. Sattva is our inner light. The purity of thoughts leads to sattvic state of mind and invokes the light of sattva. This light exuberates and gives you a radiating energy. Health, beauty and charm depend upon this energy.

The above-described three steps can lead you towards a mental state of sattva. Do these practices regularly. They take only a few minutes of your time everyday but you accumulate a priceless wealth of sattva over a period of time. It is important that you do them without any break. With the breaks, the mind begins to wander and you will have to begin from the beginning once again.

You need to make a personal effort in terms of directing your mental energies away from tamasic thoughts. With multiple efforts to attain a sattvic mental state, you will gradually get rid of nervous and tense behaviour. Tension and stress is only a mental state that we create ourselves due to lack of wisdom. Sattva gives us that wisdom. In fact, all of us have this inherent wisdom; we only need to awaken it within us. It is covered with the darkness of ignorance. Ignorance is to take too seriously the reality of the world at sensuous level and ignore the subtle capabilities of mind which lead us to the level of spirituality. Just as a dirty cloth looks beautiful after washing and sun drying, similarly sattvic thoughts give us a pure and radiant appearance.

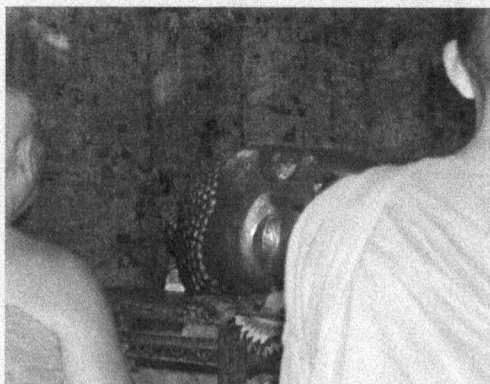

3
Care and Treatment to Enhance Beauty and Charm

This chapter has two sections. The first section is about the hygiene and care of the body and the second section is about special treatments for beautifying the skin and getting rid of various imbalances.

External care and cleansing

Care and hygiene of the body plays a very important role to maintain a youthful appearance and attractive looks. Sometimes, a little negligence gives you a shabby appearance and makes you look unattractive. The things I am going to describe below for the maintenance of different parts of the body are extremely simple and you can easily make them a part of your routine cleansing.

Care of eyes

In our appearance, eyes express the silent language of our inner being. We get familiar with the colour and form of this cosmos through our eyes. Eyes and vision are the functions of pitta energy. Care of the eyes is essential to get a bright look. Do the following for the care of your eyes:

- Upon getting up in the morning, wash your eyes with cold water. Then splash water in the open eyes with a great force.
- If you have problems with vision, do some other exercises with water. These are described later in the chapter under the section on wrinkles.
- Once a week, give your eyes bath with basil water

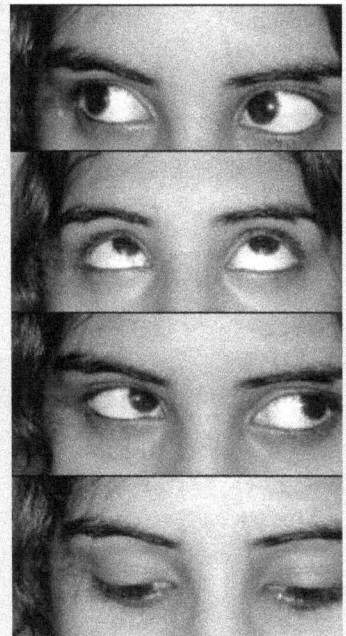

- Use some mild eye drops (Ayurvedic or homeopathic) two times a day to save your eyes from dryness and pollution.
- Do some of the following yogic exercises for the eyes:
    o Move your eyeballs in different directions. Make round movements with the eyeballs. Keep your neck and head still, move your eyeballs upwards, then on the extreme right side, then completely downwards and ultimately on the right side.
    o Concentrate on the reflection of the sun in water.
    o Concentrate on rising and setting sun.
    o Concentrate on the sun through leaves.
    o Face the sun with closed eyes and move your head gradually from left to right.

Ayursnanam (Ayurvedic bath) for the care of skin

Ayurvedic bath is different from the Western concept of taking a bath by sitting in water. It is done by putting water on you from a bucket or a source of water with the help of a small container. A shower can also serve this purpose. The Ayurvedic bath has various little practices for the rejuvenation of the body. You require putting water on your body several times. Your mental state is equally important and this bath is meant to clean the body, energise it, purify the mind, throw away bad thoughts and enhance the healing process in case of disorders.

- Wet your body with water. Rub some soap between your palms and put some sesame oil on the soap in your palms. Mix the soap and the oil by rubbing your palms together. Apply this mixture on your whole body with some force. You may have to repeat this process of mixing soap and oil several times to have enough for your entire body.
- Pour water on yourself to wash off the soap and keep rubbing your body with your hands to take out the last traces of soap.
- Let the water flow on your body and take away the entire dirt. Concentrate your thoughts on your body and wish that all the impurities from your body and mind are washed away.
- After the soap is washed away, massage your whole body with a massage brush. Pay special attention to all the joints and areas where there is more flesh like the thighs, hips and so on. Massage the neck region and the middle of the back (the place of the vertebral column) several times. It will activate and rejuvenate your body. Pour hot water on yourself after the massage and apply some warm coconut oil all over your body. Keep the coconut oil bottle in hot water as at temperatures lower than 25⁰ C,

this oil solidifies. Rub the body properly and everywhere with oil. Oil provides strength and beauty to the body and tranquillity to the mind. After you have rubbed the oil well and the body has absorbed it, pour some warm water on yourself to wash off the extra oil.

- Massage the toe of your left foot with right foot and the other way around. Similarly, massage your thumbs and press on the space between your thumb and the index finger. Finally, massage your ears by pressing the ear lobe. Take the earlobe between your thumb and fingers and press it at various points.

- Dip two fingers in mustard oil, stick them in your nostril and inhale. This will make you sneeze. Then blow your nose strongly. Finish the bath by pouring some hot water on yourself and wishing yourself a peaceful day.

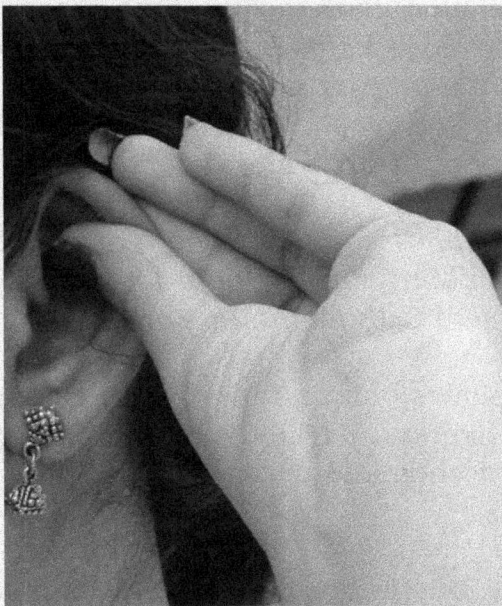

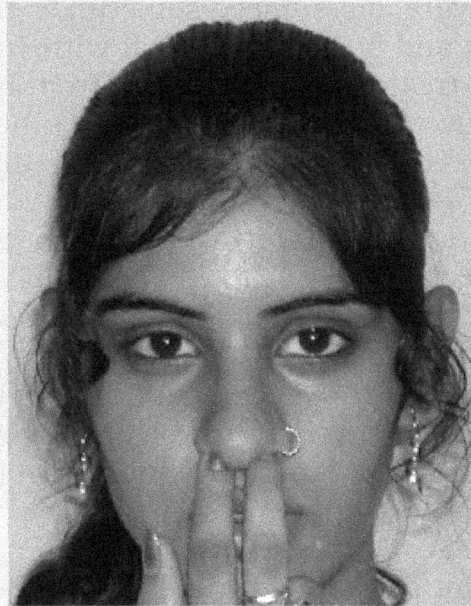

Care of hair

Oiling your hair: Head should be oiled and massaged once a week. The method to do head massage is given in the next chapter.

Washing your hair: Use mild shampoos without any nasty chemicals in them. Many shampoos dry the skin excessively or the chemicals in them irritate the skull thus resulting in dermatitis in the form of dandruff. Make sure that you wash off well after applying a shampoo so that no traces of it are left.

Ayurvedic shampoo

Traditionally in Ayurveda, a mixture of soap nuts (Ritha) and Amala are used to wash the hair. Mix the powder of these two in the ratio of 1:2 tablespoons and soak in 200 ml of water overnight. Next day, cook the decoction a little and filter it to wash your hair.

Beautifying the hair: These days, many conditioners are sold for beautifying hair. A simple home recipe is to mix a good quality vinegar with honey in a ratio of 2:1. After washing your hair, massage gently with this mixture and leave for a minute. Rinse it off.

Due to vata imbalance, sometimes the hair gives a shabby appearance. Oil massage and measures to deal with vata vikriti help. Besides that, you can give a henna treatment. Make paste from henna powder and apply on dry and clean hair. Leave for half an hour to one hour and wash it off. After this treatment, your hair will stay together properly and not fly here and there.

Pure henna does not leave colour so quickly, thus there is no fear of getting red colour on your hair with a freshly made paste and left only for an hour on the hair. You will see below that dying treatment with henna has another method.

Dying the hair: One can get different colours of hair with diverse combinations with henna. However, the variations like industrial dyes are not possible. Considering the long-term side effects of chemical dyes, it is better to stick to the natural products.

Make sure that the powdered henna you buy is pure and no dye is mixed with it. Use the following combinations for diverse colours. These colours are for grey hair or very light hair like blonde hair. The treatments given below do not make the dark hair lighter or decolour the hair.

1. **Red hair:** Take fine powder of pure henna and make its paste with hot water in a wrought iron vessel. Add a tablespoon of trifala powder for each 50 gm of henna to make a balanced preparation. Depending upon the length of your hair, you need 50 to 100 gm of henna powder. Whip well with a wooden spoon and leave the paste for 24 hours like this. Mix from time to time as the iron reacts with henna and makes it blackish. Wash your hair, comb them and dry them. Make partitions and apply henna on small locks of hairs. Apply well so that the hairs are well smeared everywhere. Tie them if you have long hair and cover them with

a plastic hood that has small holes in it. You can take a shower cap and punch some holes in it. Leave for about four hours or until dry. Wash off the henna paste with warm water and apply a mixture of vinegar and honey in the ratio of 2:1. Massage your hair with this conditioner and rinse it off in the end. Do not shampoo or use any soap at this stage.

2. **Reddish brown hair:** The method is essentially the same accept that you make this paste in a special decoction. Cook one tablespoon of black tea in about 100 ml of water for 2-3 minutes and filter it. Add a teaspoon of instant coffee into it and make the above described henna and trifala paste in this tea-coffee decoction. Leave for 24 hours in the same way and treat your hair as described above.

3. **Brown hair:** To make the tint more brown than reddish, add a tablespoon of dried and powdered shells of walnuts in the above recipe. These are used as natural dye for wool in my part of the Himalayan Mountains. In addition, add a tablespoon of amala powder to get a darker tint. Do the treatment in the same way as described above.

4. Alternatively, to get **brown hair**, you can add amala powder to recipe number 2 along with a tablespoon of bhringraj powder. Bhringraj is not available abroad and therefore you can stick to the other choice of recipes.

Combing and hairstyling: Comb your hair properly twice a day to rejuvenate the hair roots. Combing also serves as massage. Brushing alone is not sufficient. Besides combing your hair in the morning for dressing up, also comb them once again before going to bed.

Most of the men in the world and many women in the West cut their hair. In Ayurvedic texts, it is advised to make good hairstyling and in case of long hair, it is advised to brad them or tie them properly. If you have long hair, you need to trim them from time to time to ensure healthy growth. Our hairs keep falling and new ones keep growing. If you have excessive hair fall, apply sesame oil prepared with herbs (see next chapter) and make sure that your pitta is balanced.

Prevention of dandruff: Many people seem to complain about dandruff. As I have described above, this form of scaling of the skin seems to be an allergic reaction due to some irritants that may be coming from some shampoos or washing powders you use or from some fabric. Observe carefully the factors that cause dandruff in your particular case and avoid them. Besides that, try one of the following measures to get rid of dandruff.

- Application of oil once a week is extremely essential. Extreme dryness can give rise to dandruff. Add 10% neem oil into coconut oil and apply that on your scalp. Leave for a day or overnight and wash it off. If you feel better repeat every week until the problem is completely eradicated.
- Take fine powder of trifala*. To make the powder very fine, pass it from a muslin cloth or extra fine strainer that is used in India to make white flour (maida) from normal whole-wheat flour (atta). Mix two tablespoon of this powder into two tablespoons of warm ghee to make a paste. Apply this on the scalp and leave it there for several hours.
- Make a paste of fine powder of liquorice with ghee in the similar manner as described above. Apply on the scalp and leave for several hours before rinsing it off.
- Make a mixture of limejuice, coconut oil and honey in equal quantity. Apply it on scalp and leave there for about half an hour and wash it off.

Care of hands and feet

Our feet carry the burden of our body and our hands are always hyperactive to perform all kinds of functions. Hands are always exposed to air. Both hands and feet are vulnerable to vata imbalance because of their functions related to movements. Therefore they need special care. In fact, the symptoms of vata imbalance anywhere in the body show on these extremities of our body. That is why hand and feet massage of specific points is an important part of the North Indian Ayurvedic massage. Pressing and massage as well as special oil bath for hands and feet are described in the next chapter. Here are some points you should pay attention to for the care of your hands and feet.

- Nail should be well cut every 8 to 10 days. While cutting the nails, take special care to cut them well from the corners so that they do not grow in your skin.
- Clean the nails with a brush while bathing and rub the sole of the feet with pumice stone or something similar. Feet develop some hard skin and gentle rubbing can remove this skin.

Cracked heels: Some people get hard and rough skin on their heels and get cracks. Normally this happens in hot countries. Apply liquorice paste with ghee as has been described above in case of dandruff. Alternatively, apply a thick layer of Vaseline and put on socks. Repeat this several time until cured.

---

* Trifala is a mixture of three Ayurvedic fruits in equal quantity. Amala, Harad and Baheda are taken without their stones, dried, weighed in equal quantity and powdered. Trifala can be bought readymade and is also available abroad. Take care to read the date. Plant products lose their medicinal value if old.

Excessive hair on the body

Many women use drastic methods like hot wax to remove extra hairs from their face or arms and legs. Some people also use hair-removing creams. These methods are too nasty for the skin and should not be used. Try to remove the hairs in an appropriate manner without causing shock to your body.

Facial hairs including the eyebrows should be removed one by one with a pair of good tweezers or forceps. Besides that, rub roughly ground powder of black gram with some ghee and water in it on the facial hairs to weaken them. Hairs on arms and legs can also be gradually rubbed with the same paste to weaken them. In fact this paste is used to remove hairs from the bodies of the babies if they are born with excessive hair. It is specially done for baby girls.

Use pumice stone to remove extra hairs from arms and legs. Always rub after bath and after applying oil. Keep wetting the body while rubbing with pumice stone gently. Do not try to remove all the hairs at once as that will require too much rubbing and that harms the upper layer of the skin. Removing hairs with gradual rubbing weaken their roots and growth diminishes considerably over a period of time.

Underarms and pubic hairs can be removed with a razor. Always apply some coconut oil after removing the hairs from these places.

Beautifying your Appearance

I will give you the recipes of various treatments for improving the quality of your skin and complexion, and enhancing radiance. However, you will have to make a selection according to your requirement. Some people suffer from dry skin whereas there are others who have fatty and oily skin. Generally, people of kapha prakriti have good and smooth skin. You should keep in mind that the aim of Ayurvedic applications is not only to remove the symptoms but also to replace imbalance with balance and harmony. The whole system should be rejuvenated and strengthened in order to function in an optimum manner.

Oily and fatty skin

People with oily and fatty skin make the mistake of using too much soap and shampoo and ultimately this has a contrary effect. The scientific reason for this is that our skin and scalp secrete oils as means of protection. If you wash too much, the already active glands become even more active as a protection mechanism. You get trapped in a vicious cycle. I know many people who shampoo their hair several times a week due to the problem of oily and fatty hair and finally get many problems with the scalp. The cause of fatty and oily skin according to Ayurveda is the vitiation of pitta. There is too much heat in the body and one needs to take diet that is cold in its Ayurvedic nature to balance the body fire in general. Various anointing are needed to balance the excessive heat in those particular parts of the body.

Dry skin

Persons with dry skin have generally an under function of secreting glands. The skin has to be massaged regularly with various kinds of oils to revive the proper functioning of the glands. This happens due to vata vitiation and the balance is created by oil massage and some warm measures.

Five weeks treatment for oily skin

You may have the problem of oily skin in one particular part of the body or all over. The external treatments should be applied accordingly. Many people are only bothered about their face and ignore the rest of the body. Do not ignore any part of your body and apply this treatment either on the whole body or on excessively oily parts. Oily feet may stink. If you have an oily back, you may get some itching or pimples.

First Week
1. Wash well the affected part with warm water. Avoid using soap. Clean with fresh (uncooked) milk or make some paste of besin (chickpea flour) with fresh milk and rub that on the skin to remove excessive fat. Dry well by wiping gently with a towel.
2. Apply a thin paste of yellow earth (*multani mitti*). Let it dry and wash it off with cold water.
3. Massage the skin strongly with coconut oil for about five minutes. Soak a towel in the hot water, squeeze it and wipe off the excessive fat.

Second week
1. The step one is same as for the first week.

2. Apply sandalwood paste. Make the paste by rubbing sandalwood on a stone with some water. Keep the paste for at least 15 minutes and then wash it off.

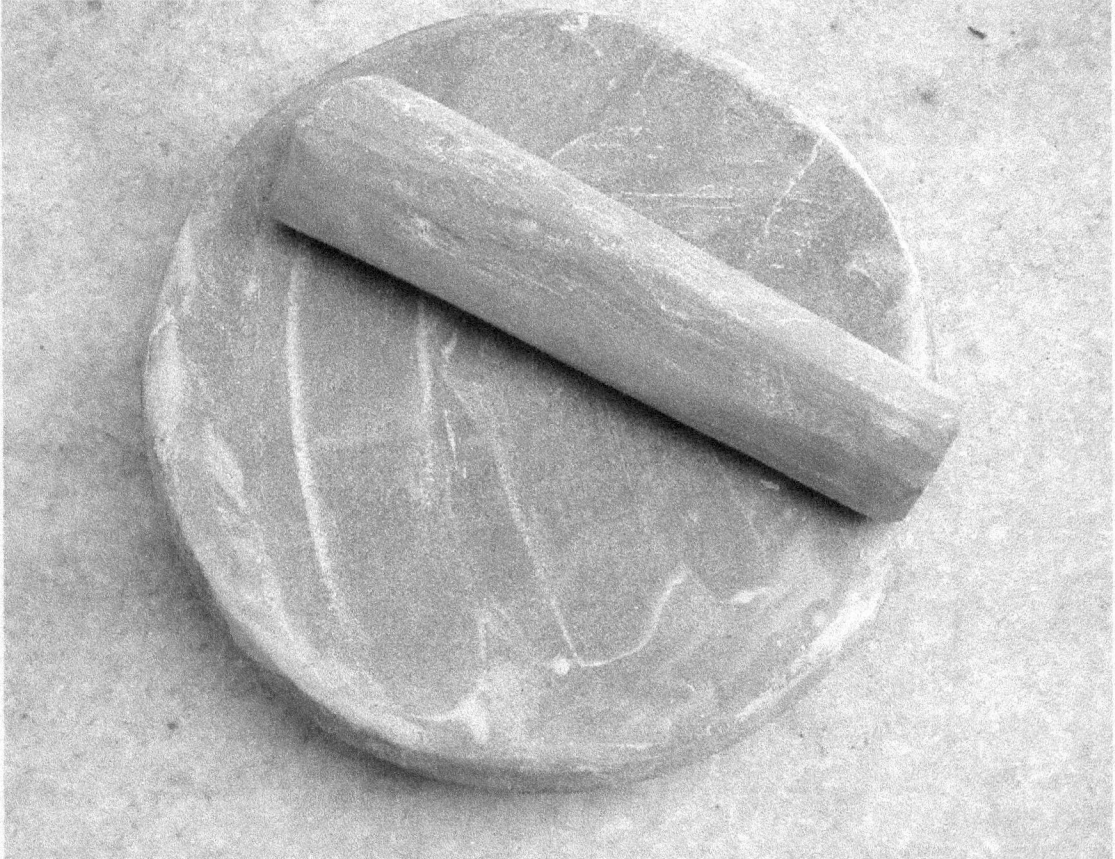

3. Massage strongly with milk skin for five minutes and wash off the excessive fat with a warm and wet towel as described above.

Third week
1. Wash the affected part as you did for the previous two weeks. However, if you feel that your skin is better than before, you may simply wash with warm water and dry.
2. Apply the pulp of *Aloe vera*. This covers the skin like a mask. Leave it as long as you can but at least for 15 minutes before washing or peeling it off.
3. Massage strongly with milk skin for five minutes and wash off the excessive fat with a warm and wet towel as described above.

Fourth week
1. Wash the skin with warm water and dry it properly.

2. Make a thick paste of powdered shirish* seeds with water and apply on the skin. Leave it until it dries up.
3. Wash off this mask after about half an hour and massage with warm ghee. Wash with warm water to get rid of the fat.

Fifth week

1. Wash your skin with warm water and dry it well.
2. Apply a mask of *ubtan*.

UBTAN RECIPE

Chickpea flour (basin)	3 tablespoons
Curcuma (haldi)	½ teaspoon
Sandalwood paste	1 teaspoon
Mustard oil	2 teaspoons
Shirish powder or powdered pomegranate peels	1 teaspoon
Sesame paste or oil	1 tablespoon

Mix all the ingredients well to make a paste. If the paste is too thick, you can add some spoons of milk or water. Apply the ubtan on the skin and leave the mask until it dries up. Gently rub to take it off. Wash with warm water.

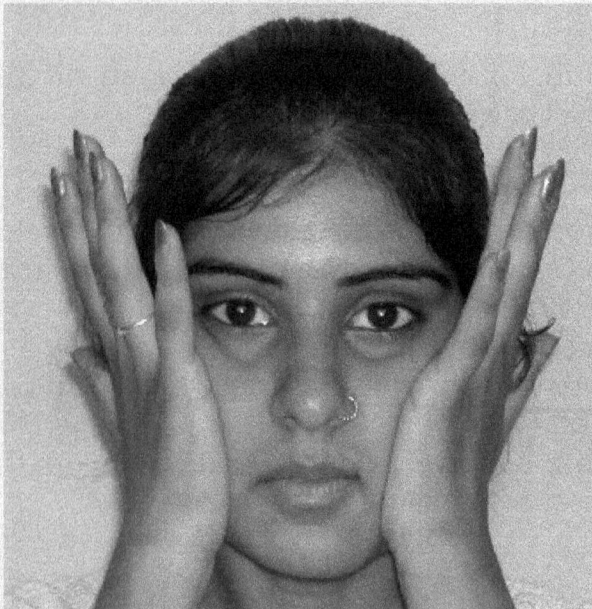

Five weeks treatment for dry skin

First Week

1. Give a vigorous massage with coconut oil.
2. Give vapour treatment on the affected parts.
3. Wipe off gently with a towel.
4. Anoint with milk skin and leave it as long as you can but at least 15 minutes.
5. Wash with warm water or wet and hot towel. Do not use any soap or any cream later on.

---

* If shirish seeds are not available, use dried and powdered orange peels or pomegranate peels.

Second week

1. Give vigorous massage with olive oil or sesame oil.
2. Give vapour treatment.
3. Dry and anoint with sandalwood paste.
4. Wash off the sandalwood paste after it dries up and dry with a towel.
5. Apply warm ghee and massage well.
6. Wipe with hot and warm towel after 15 minutes or more.

Third week

1. Give vigorous massage with almond oil.
2. Give vapour treatment.
3. Apply the pulp of *Aloe vera* and leave it as long as you can but at least for 15 minutes.
4. Wash and dry and apply milk. Wipe it gently with warm and wet towel.

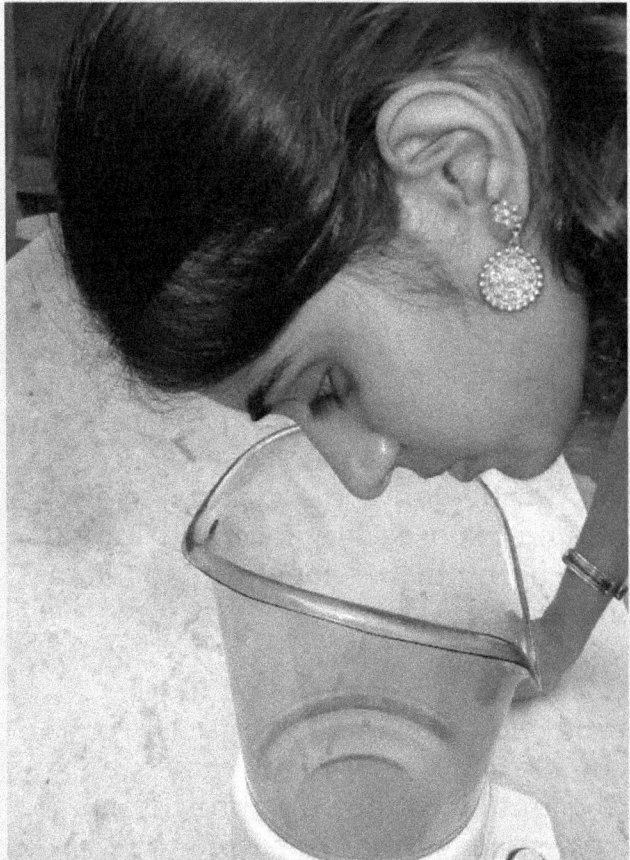

Fourth week

1. Apply a thin mask of chiranji paste made with milk. (Chiranji is a nut. See Chapter 8 for more details).
2. Let the mask dry and gradually rub to take off the mask.
3. Wipe gently with a warm and wet towel

Fifth week

1. Make a paste of chiranji and peeled almonds in equal quantities and mix it with some red sandalwood paste. Apply this as a protective cream or a thin mask and wipe off with a warm and

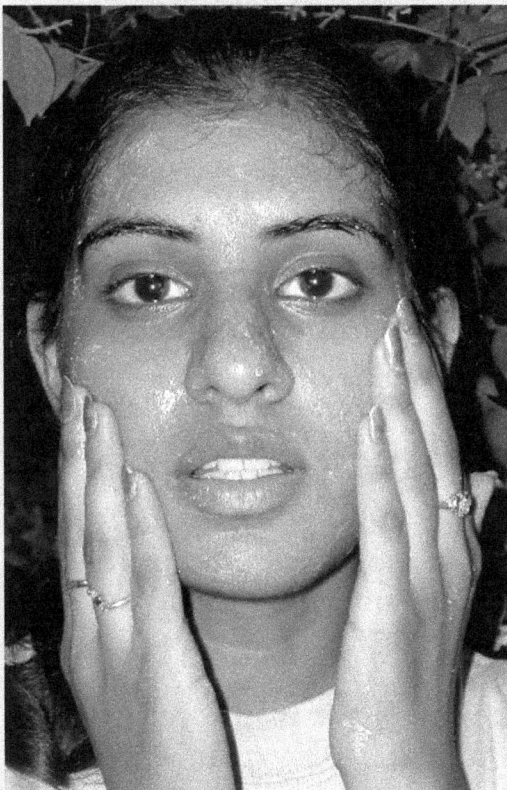

wet towel.
2. You can even continue to use it after the 5 weeks treatment is over.

Care of the normal skin

Even if you think that your skin is neither dry nor oily, it is smooth and fine, you still need to care about it to keep it nice for a long time. Take the treatment of third to fifth week described above for the treatment of dry skin. Skin in general is vulnerable to vata as it is exposed to air. Particularly those parts, which remain exposed like face and hands are even more sensitive to vata imbalance.

Coconut is a wonderful oil for the protection of skin and getting a good complexion. Use it regularly.
Coconut oil is known to protect us from sunrays and thus from the ultraviolet radiations.

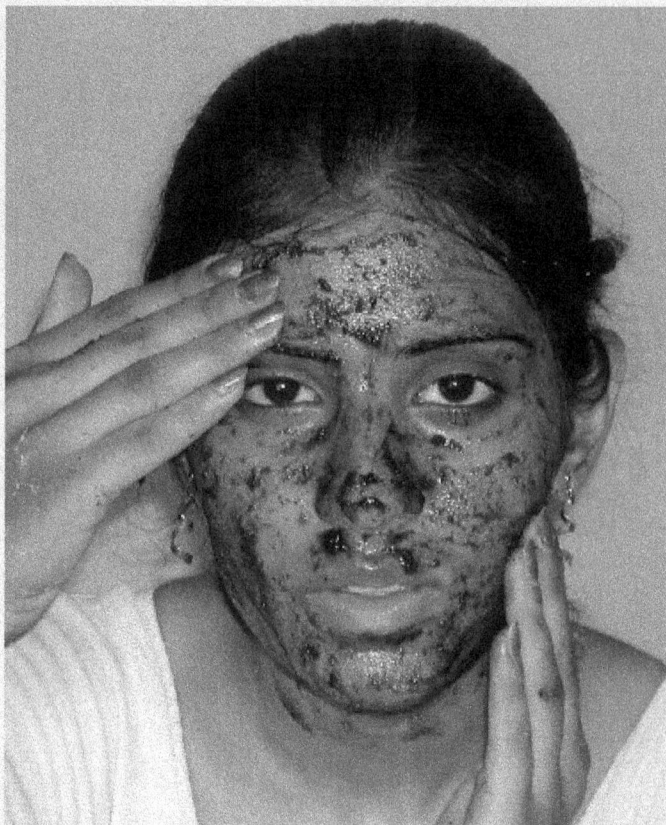

Special treatment and care

From time to time, you should give yourself special treatment for the care of your skin and to make your 'outer shell' stronger in today's polluted environment. I give below three recipes. Make the preparation and use it while bathing. Do not use any soap or oil when you give yourself one of these treatments. Rub the preparation with your hand on your wet body. Take each time some of it on your palm and keep rubbing different parts of your body with it. Wash it off with warm water in the end.

Milk and honey bath: Take ¼ litre of full milk, if possible fresh and untreated. Heat it a little to make it warm. Add 2 tablespoons of honey into it and mix well. Use it as described above for bathing.

Cream-honey bath: Take fresh untreated milk and put it in the refrigerator. When it is cold, its cream will gather on the top. Take this cream and mix it with equal quantity of honey and whip them together. Use this preparation as described above.

Pranchamrit snanam (the bath with five nectars or the bath of gods): This is a very special preparation with several things in it and is good for all types of skin. It has a very healing effect on the skin and people with skin problems should use it often. In the rituals for bathing gods in the temples, all these five components are taken. That is why I have called it the bath of gods. However, for the gods, these components are taken one by one whereas you will use them mixed in the form of a creamy paste.

Pancha means five and amrit means nectar. Take following five components and mix them well.

- Ghee,
- Cream,
- Honey,
- Sesame oil
- Sandalwood paste

Take three tablespoons each of first four components and one tablespoon of the sandalwood paste. Heat the ghee to melt it and add oil in it. Mix well and add cream and honey. Cream should be obtained from the fresh, untreated milk or take the milk skin. Add sandalwood paste in the end. Mix all components well with a hand mixer to obtain a creamy, homogenous paste. Rub it on your entire body, leave it for a while and then wash with warm water. Your skin will feel smooth like a baby after taking the bath of gods. You can use this mixture as body or face cream for everyday use. But you need to rinse it off with warm water.

Prevention and treatment of wrinkles

Skin looses its elasticity with age and we get wrinkles. Cause of wrinkles is of course aging but some people get them more and some less. Some get them too early and the others late and less. It is important that you understand the factors that cause wrinkles and make a multidimensional effort to avoid them the longest possible.

Besides aging, wrinkles are caused due to the following factors:

- Excessive dryness in the body (vata imbalance)

- Excessive heat in the body (pitta imbalance)
- Lack of appropriate rest and sleep
- Regular intake of alcohol and tobacco
- Excessive physical activity
- Lack of physical activity
- Excessive use of senses, like talking too much, too loud and so on
- Gaining and losing weight frequently without proper oil saturation

I give under this subtitle some specific exercises for preventing wrinkles but this whole book is oriented towards that. Oil treatments are extremely important and next chapter is exclusively devoted to that. Similarly nutrition plays a very important part. It is also essential to do fat therapy from time to time. I have named it as 'the inner lubrication of the body' and it is described later in this Chapter. Besides what is given below, other precautions given in this book are also essential to prevent wrinkles.

Here are some exercises to activate the skin and muscles to prevent and delay the formation of wrinkles. The existing wrinkles can be reduced and smoothened with these exercises and with some treatments. Devote few minutes everyday to do the exercises described below.

Exercises to maintain the facial elasticity: Our face has a complicated musculature. Muscles of the upper and lower lips are horizontal to the mouth. From both sides of the mouth, three different muscles originate in three different directions. They go to upper and middle cheek and the chin. It is essential to enhance their elasticity by diverse exercises to hinder the facial wrinkles.

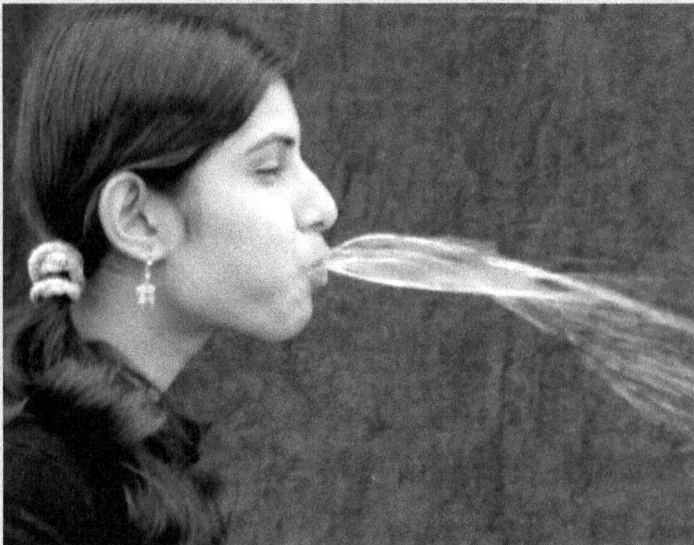

Fill your mouth with water and throw it gradually as far as you can. Repeat this 6-7 times and do this exercise twice a day.

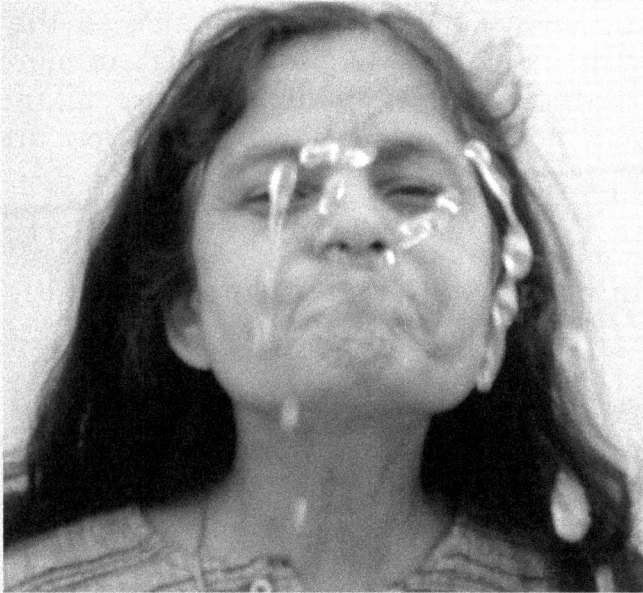

Take some water in your mouth. Project your lower lip outwards and throw the water upwards towards your eyes with force. This water should go inside your nose and eyes. It will take you some time to attain perfection in doing this exercise. Repeat it 4-5 times.

Fill your mouth with water and take it in diverse parts of the mouth with little force. Push it under the upper lip and keep it like this for few seconds.

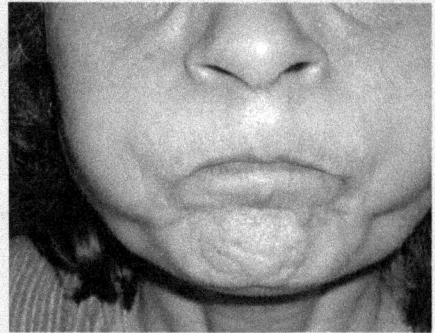

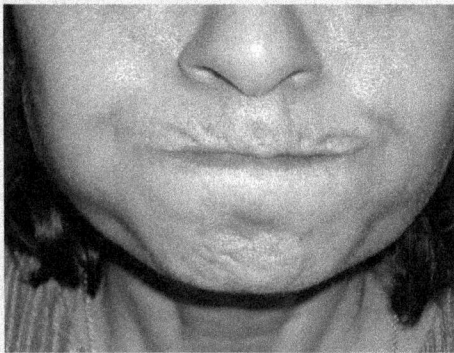

Then move it down under the lower lip and do the same. Move the water vigorously from left to right side and vice versa for few times. You can repeat these exercises during the day without water. Fill your mouth with air and do the same way.

There are some other exercises which are done without filling the mouth with water and you can do them any time of the day.

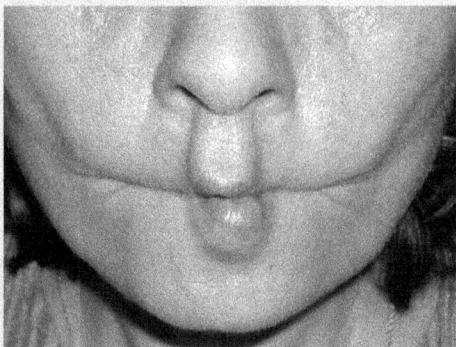

Invert your cheeks inside your mouth so that your lips make a shape like a beak. Try to move your lips up and down while they are in the shape of a beak in such a way as if you are talking with your lips.

In the same posture of beak as described above, stick your chin forward and backward several times.

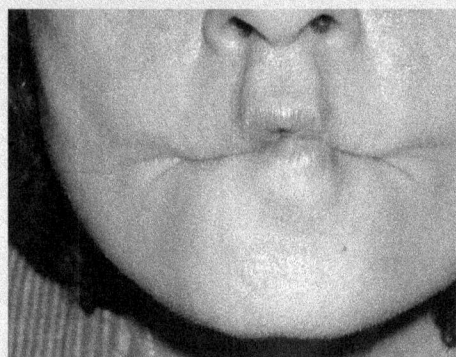

Fill your lungs with air while standing. Curl your lips and throw the air out very slowly and smoothly with a whistling noise. Empty out your lungs completely. Inhale again and repeat this exercise several times.

Maintaining the elasticity of the skin with oil treatments and massage: A regular oil treatment should be given to the body (see next chapter). It is very important that if you are dieting to lose weight, you take special care to saturate your body with coconut oily twice a week. Otherwise you will get stretch marks[*]. Pregnant women can forget about all the expensive stretch mark removing industrial creams and apply simply pure and warm coconut oil everyday. Similarly, the coconut oil treatment can gradually reduce the tissue drainage and the white marks left due to that. Many women tend to get these marks on their thighs with aging.

Enhancing facial glow and strength with pranayama (kapalbhati): This practice of pranayama is done in a sitting posture. Breathe in such a manner as if you have been running. When we run, we get breathless and we breathe through mouth and nose both altering quite spontaneously. Our system makes best of its effort to send the maximum prana energy inside. Our breathing runs very fast. Thus, in kapalbhati pranayama, you are imitating the situation of running or the breathing pattern we adopt in a situation when we are

---

[*] For more details on this theme, refer to my book: *Losing Weight with Yoga and Ayurveda*, available at www.amazon.com

breathless. After about half a minute, stop breathing like this. You will reach a state of stillness and for few seconds, you will not breathe. This practice brings a glow on your face and makes you feel good. You can repeat it for two to three times.

Caution: If you are unwell or have fever, do not do this practice. Women during menstruation should also not do this practice. In case this practice makes you feel giddy, stop immediately.

'Inner lubrication' of the body: As has been described in the previous chapter, the inner dryness is caused due to vata imbalance and it shows on your outward appearance. In this case, besides external application of oil, you also need internal lubrication. I describe below, two different modes of internal lubrication.

1. Fat treatment: This treatment is very simple and comprises of drinking ghee (fat from butter) for the following three days before going to bed in the doses given below. Whip the ghee in some hot milk along with some candy sugar. If you do not drink milk, have the ghee in a clear vegetable soup.

Day 1: Three teaspoons
Day 2: Five teaspoons
Day 3: Eight teaspoons

Caution: *Fat or obese persons or those with vitiation of kapha and pregnant women should not do this treatment.*

2. Matra basti: Basti is enema and matra basti is to introduce the fat in very small doses through anal opening. This treatment is very simple and very effective for giving you a good complexion. Persons with weak digestion may have problems with the fat intake, thus they should use matra basti. I suggest doing matra basti once a week for general well being. You can do it after finishing your bath. In case you feel dryness and have symptoms like dry throat and dry skin, you should do this treatment everyday for a week.

Matra basti should be done about an hour or more after evacuation. Buy a 5 ml syringe and use it without needle. Fill warm coconut oil or ghee into it and insert it in the anal opening. Press the syringe to put the oil in. Insert between 10 to 30 ml of oil depending on your body weight. For example, persons weighing around 75 Kg should use 30 ml. Persons weighing 50-60 kg should use 20 ml. Use only 5 ml for children between 5 to 10 years.

You can also use sesame oil or olive oil but persons with pitta vikriti should not use oil. Persons who are over-weight or have kapha vikriti should not do matra basti.

Heat balancing for good complexion

Pitta imbalance gives rise to excessively reddish complexion or pimples or skin eruptions etc. In case the measures described for pitta balance do not show their effect, take the purgation treatment to regulate your system.

Purgation: Before doing purgation, prepare your body for it by doing an oil saturating massage and fomentation (see next chapter). Take a mild purgative before going to bed. Usually in each country people know about some plant purgatives. The recommended mild purgatives in Ayurveda are the following:

1. Powdered leaves of sanaye (*Cassia agustifolia*), dose: I teaspoon with warm water.
2. Amaltas (*Cassia fistula*), Pulp from the dried beans of this tree should be taken out. Take out pulp from about 5 inches of bean, boil it in little water, filter it and drink it before going to bed.

The effect of the purgative remains about half a day. Take light, warm and fluid meals like soup or preparation of rice with vegetables for the next two days.

After this purification practice, take care that you avoid eating foods with excessive pitta energy and make your meals balanced.

Getting rid of the excessive earthy energy for a bright complexion

Jaladhauti: Kapha imbalance gives one a dull and sleepy appearance. Normally, it is possible to change it with appropriate nutrition as described in Chapter 5. Besides that, I suggest doing a simple yogic practice called jaladhauti. This practice should be done empty stomach in the morning. You will need to drink about ¾ litre of water with a pinch of rock salt in it. Bend your torso at 45^0 and throw this water out by tickling your throat with your finger. Do this practice 3-4 times in a period of two weeks. In a healthy person the vomited out water should be just as you drank it.

Wet-heat treatment: This method is quickly effective to bring you out from a dull and sleepy appearance. Take some hot water in a container and add some balm (Tiger balm, Amritanjan balm) or a similar mixture of some etheric oils available in the market. Wet some medium sized towels in this water, squeeze them and wrap them around your body. Go on changing the hot towels and do this treatment for about 15 minutes. You will need to add some hot water into the container a few times. Make sure that your towels are pleasantly warm. Close all the windows so that there is no air draft. The wet heat and the vapours from etheric oils will activate your system and have an immediate effect on your appearance. Wrap yourself well in a bathrobe and rest for about 15 minutes in warm bed (with hot water bottle) after this treatment.

Detoxification for a smooth skin

We all need to purify our blood from time to time; specially in our times with all the pesticides and preservatives we consume with our food. The toxins can harm both the inner organs as well as our skin. Detoxification gives you better skin and better complexion. Here is a simple home remedy for it.

Blood Purifier

Kalonji	10 gm
Cress seeds (chansoor)	10 gm
Ajwain	10 gm
Fenugreek seeds (methi)	10 gm
Cassia absus (chaksu)	10 gm
Basil leaves (Tulsi)	10 gm
Neem leaves	10 gm
Liquorice (mullathi)	30 gm

Take dried ingredients and powder them with the help of a small spice grinder or a coffee grinder. Mix them properly and pass it through a fine strainer. If there still are big pieces left on the strainer, grind them again. Pass this also through the strainer and throw away the leftovers. Mix the powder well with a spoon and keep it in a tightly closed jar.

Intake of the blood purifier: Take half a teaspoon of the above preparation daily for 15 days. Put the powder in your mouth and swallow it with water. It is bitter and may be unpleasant for some of you. You can eat something sweet afterwards to get rid of the bitter taste from your mouth.

If you are suffering from excessive heat or skin eruptions, too much sweating, bad smell from the body or other effects of pitta vitiation, you may continue to take the blood purifier for 30 days.

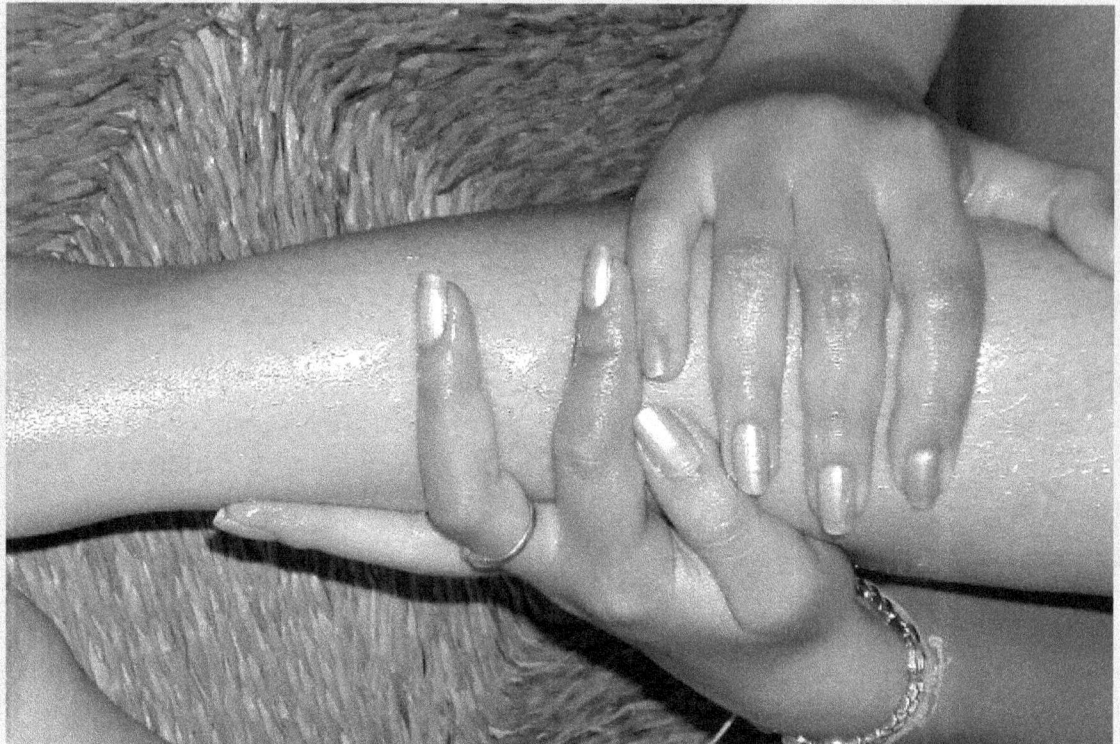

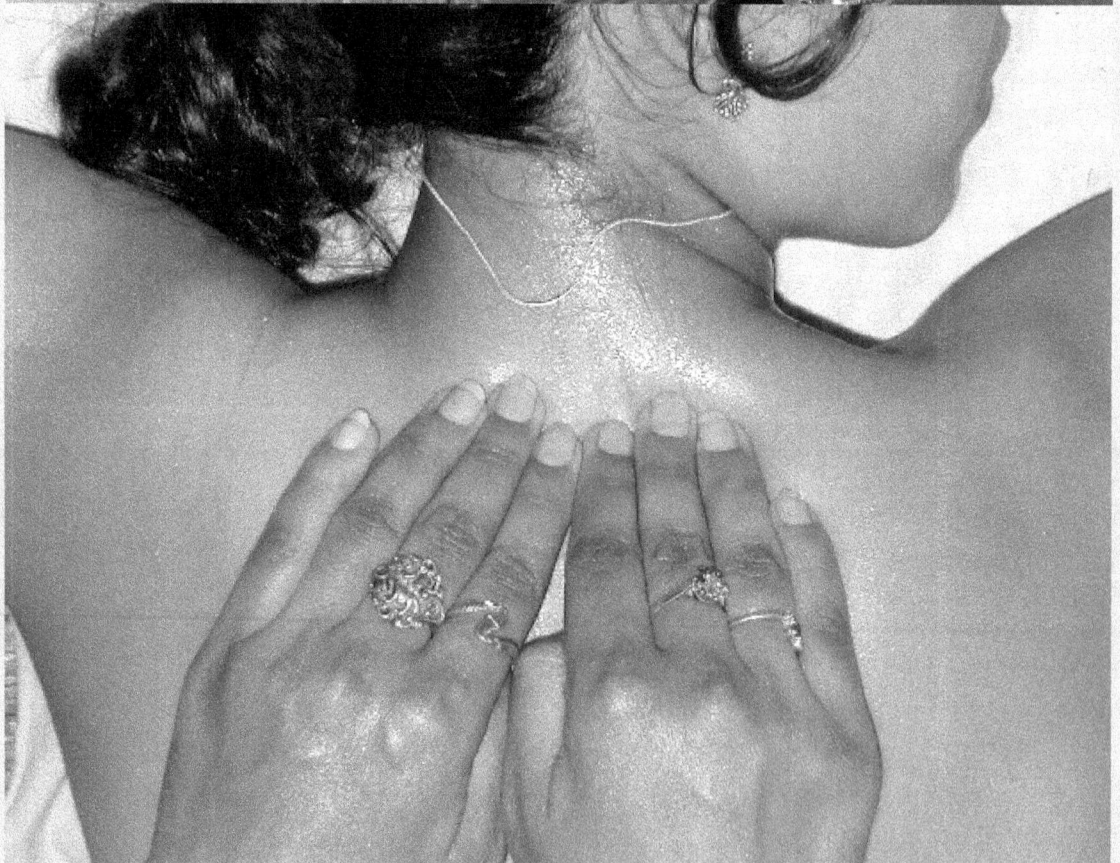

4

Oil Treatments, Massage Anointing and Fomentation

Ayurvedic external treatments with oils and different kinds of massages*, as well as fomentation or sweat therapy are highly effective in enhancing beauty and strength. The diverse anointing and oil treatments are also used to create a balance of three energies of the body. Fomentation or sweat therapy is recommended after oil treatment or massage. Many big hotels around the world are doing roaring business by offering these popular Ayurvedic treatments to people. In fact, you are made to think at such places that this is for the purification (panchakarma) and beautification of the body and that is all about Ayurveda. Some also advertised for selling these treatments as "maharajas' treatments made possible for all". In any case, in this chapter, I am going to give you simple methods, which you can do on your own or with family or friends' circle.

Oil treatments

Oil treatments are strength promoting; make the skin beautiful and resistant to infections and shocks. The great sage of Ayurveda, Charaka described the importance of the oil treatments extensively. I give some citations below from Charaka Samhita, written between 600 to 700 BC to make you aware of this ancient wisdom.

> **'As a pitcher by moistening and an axis of a wheel with lubrication become strong and jerk resistant, so by oil application, the body becomes firm, smooth skinned, free from disturbances of vata and tolerant to physical exercise and exertion.**
> **Vayu (vata) is predominant in tactile sense organs which is located in the skin. Thus, oil application is the most beneficial for skin and should be done regularly.**

---

* This chapter tells you the very fundamental, do-it-yourself massage methods. I am preparing a separate book with the details of the North Indian Ayurvedic massage methods for healing.

> **Those who do a regular application of oil on the body do not become much affected due to accidental injuries or strenuous work. With daily application of oil on the body, a person is endowed with pleasant touch, trimmed body parts and becomes strong charming and less affected with old age.**
> **Rubbing the body (with oil), alleviates foul smell, heaviness, drowsiness, itching, dirt, anorexia and excessive sweat'**[1]

Charaka further describes various benefits of oil saturation on diverse parts of the body.

> **Head:**
> **'One who moistens his head with unctuous substances does not suffer from headache, hair fall, baldness and greying of hair. A regular application of oil on head makes the hair firmly rooted, long and shiny and the skull is strengthened. The senses become strong; one gets sound sleep and feels happy. The face becomes cheerful and gets a pleasant glow.'**[2]
> **Ears:**
> **'By saturating ears with oil daily, ear diseases due to vata, stiff neck and jaws, hard of hearing and deafness do not occur.'**[3]
> **Feet:**
> **'By saturating feet with oil, coarseness, stiffness, roughness, fatigue and numbness of feet are alleviated. One gets delicacy, strength and firmness in feet. Clarity in vision is attained and vata is pacified. A regular oil massage on feet is preventive against sciatica, cracking of soles, and constrictions of veins and ligaments.'**[4]

You can do the oil massages and oil treatments given below at home without much hassle.

Weekly oil saturating self-massage[*]
More than twenty-five years ago, while studying Charaka Samhita, I was extremely impressed with the above description. I was living in Germany and it was not possible to get a masseuse at home like it used to be in my family during my childhood. I developed methods of doing this massage on my own and saturating my body with oil regularly, at least once a week. In fact, it was

---

[1] Charaka Samhita, Sutrasthana, V, 85-89, 93
[2] *Ibid*, 81-83
[3] *Ibid*, 84
[4] *Ibid*, 90-92
[*] For more details of this massage with photographs, consult my book- Programming your Life with Ayurveda.

more or less a part of research for me at that time and the results were amazing. Later, I started teaching these techniques of self-massage in my Ayurvedic weekend classes. I describe below the various steps of this oil-saturating self-massage and later, I will discuss about the choice of oil.

- Choose a warm corner of your house if it is cold weather. Take some warm oil and start applying with your right hand on your left hand. After applying on each finger and on both sides of your hand, massage the hand with pressure. Massage individually each finger.
- Apply the oil on whole arm in long and strong stokes. Apply oil also on your shoulder and underarm. Go on massaging so that the oil gets absorbed. Keep applying more oil if needed. Different people need different quantity of oil depending upon their prakriti or state of vikriti.
- Repeat the same with your left hand on your right hand and arm.
- Massage with plenty of oil your left foot. Use both your hands. Apply oil on the lower leg with long stokes and applying good pressure so that the oil is absorbed. Similarly massage the whole leg and subsequently repeat the same on right foot and leg.
- Stand up and apply oil on your buttocks and both the sides of your torso. Apply pressure to get the oil absorbed.
- Sit down again and apply oil on front part of your body, neck and face by the application of oil and massage strokes several times.
- Apply oil on your lower back by extending your arms behind and on upper back by taking your arms from above. In case you have problems, take a plastic sheet, smear oil on it and role with your back on it.
- To saturate the body completely, repeat the whole process two more times.

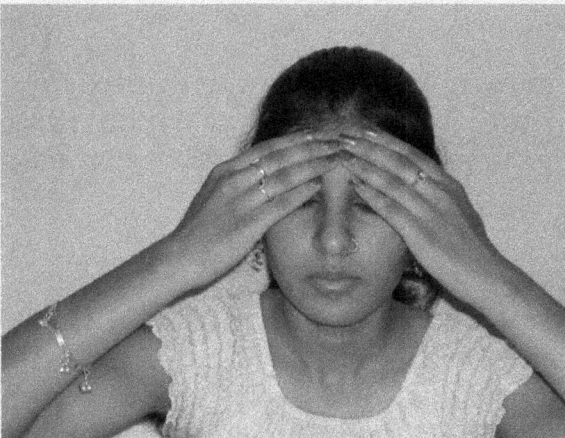

Face massage
For invigorating your face, massage it at least once a week with the palms of your hands after the oil application. Make vigorous and round movements with both your palms on both sides of the face simultaneously.

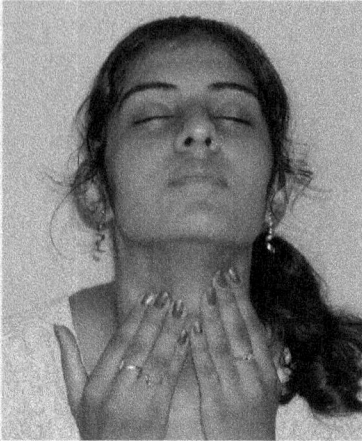

Massage inwards under the chin and downwards on the neck region with your fingers. Massage your forehead by moving the fingers of both your hands in opposite direction. For attaining a bright and attractive face, you can do this massage daily before your bath.

Head massage

For acquiring an attractive and glamorous appearance, you need to have good and healthy hair. Most people get fascinated by television advertisements of various shampoos to get good hair and end up having problems of dryness and dandruff. Like other parts of the body, our scalp needs oiling and massage regularly. In Ayurveda, it is believed that nourishing the roots of the hairs with oil is very important. Take some oil in a plate, smear your

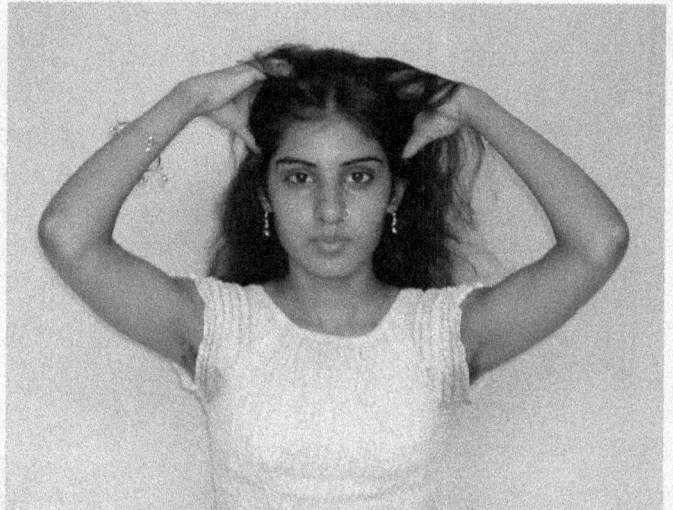

fingertips in it and apply on your scalp by moving your fingers with pressure. Apply on each and every part of the scalp and repeat the application three times. Pay special attention of massaging the area around and above the ears and massage also the earlobes.

Choice of oil

Those who suffer from very dry skin should use coconut oil for several weeks until their body becomes smooth and does not get dry everyday. Later, you can also use other oils like olive, sesame and almond alternatively. Persons with imbalance of pitta and having very red complexion and hot skin should use only coconut oil or ghee.

Ayurvedic Beauty Oil

Ingredients:

Liquorice	100 gm
Cloves	25 gm
Cardamom	10 gm
Nutmeg	25 gm
Essentials oils of	10 ml each
Fennel	
Jasmine	
Rose	
Ghee or sesame oil or olive oil	300 gm

Powder the first four ingredients. Heat the oil or ghee at a very high temperature in a big pot. You need a very big pot because you are going to add powdered spices into very hot oil and it boils over with great force. Before putting the spices, remove the hot oil from the stove and add the spices gradually. Once you have added the spices, heat at a low fire for few minutes. Leave it like this overnight. Filter the oil through a muslin cloth by squeezing well so that you can remove all the oil. You will obtain about 200 ml of oil. Separately, mix all the essential oils and leave them like this for a week. Shake this mixture few times a day. After a week, mixed these essential oils into your other preparation and shake the bottle well.

Ayurvedic Hair Oil

Use the following ingredients to make Ayurvedic hair oil for half litre sesame oil. The method of preparing the oil is the same as above.

Brahmi	100 gm
Trifala	50 gm
Amala	50 gm
Liquorice	50 gm

In case you do not have Ayurvedic hair oil, use coconut, olive, almond or any other nut oil or simply sesame oil.

After the oil massage

It is important to keep the oil on the body for some time. Before dressing up, you remove excessive oil from your body either by rubbing some chickpea flour (*basin*) on your body or simply with a warm and wet towel. A wet fomentation is recommended after a few hours of massage. This can be done in a normal bathtub at home.

Wet fomentation

In Ayurveda, fomentation or perspiration therapy is of two kinds– dry and wet. Dry consists of sweating in dry and hot place (like a sauna) and wet is like a vapour bath. However, in Ayurveda, exposing to cold or air is strictly forbidden after fomentation therapy. I describe below a simple method to do wet fomentation at home.

- Before your bath, make sure that you close all the windows and the place should be warm. Prepare your bed and make it warm with a hot water bottle. Make some ginger + basil + cardamom + pepper tea in a thermos and keep it besides your bed.
- Prepare a hot bath. Add some drops of essential oils like rose, jasmine, fennel or their combination into it. Sit in the bath comfortably and make sure that the water remains hot. Add more hot water from time to time.
- When you start sweating, come out of your bath, put on a bathrobe and go to your warm bed. Take some tea and rest. You will continue to sweat for a while.
- Rest for about ½ an hour after you have stopped sweating.

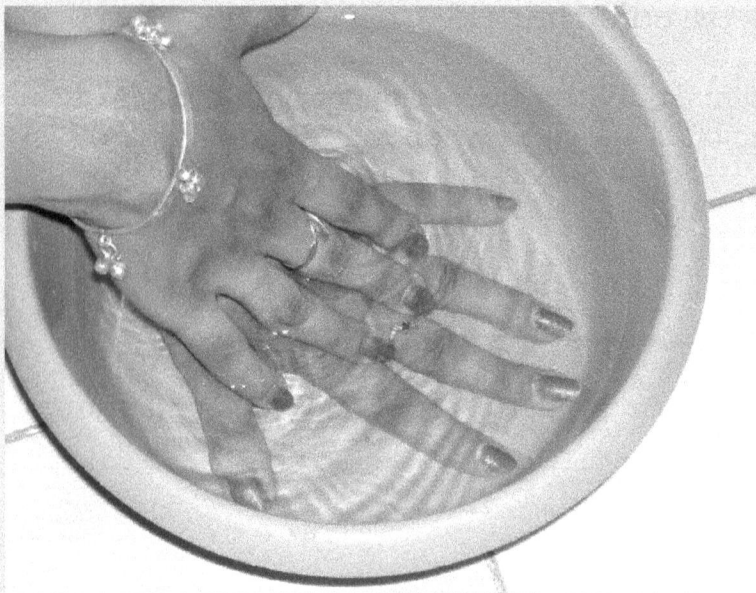

Tail snanam (oil bath) for individual parts of the body

Hands and feet are the most active parts of our body and need special treatment. Sensitive to vata due to their activities and exposure, I suggest doing special protective treatments for them. Similarly, our abdomen is the central point of the body and oil treatment of this region has a calming effect on internal organs for pacifying the disturbed doshas.

Kara snanam (oil bath for hands)

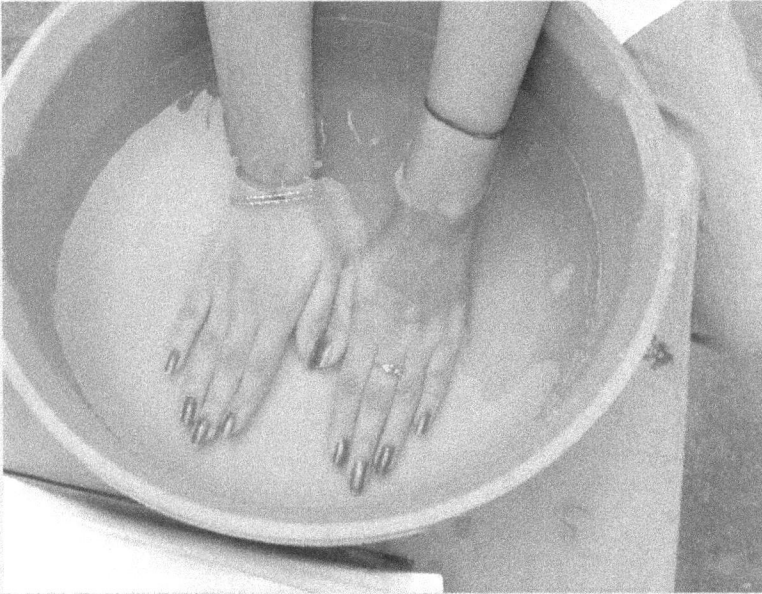

Take sesame or olive oil for this treatment. You can also use Ayurvedic beauty oil described earlier. Warm it and put it in a small plastic container in which you can dip both your hands comfortably. Keep the hands still for few minutes. Then rub and press them with each other. Keep them as long as you can in the oil bath. At least fifteen minutes are recommended. Take them out carefully and let all the oil drip in the container. Give them vapour treatment above a pot of boiling water for few minutes. Wrap them in a towel and rest for 15 minutes.

This treatment will give relaxing feeling not only to your hands but also to your whole body. Hands will look soft and beautiful. The oil used here can be kept for the oil treatment of feet.

Pada snanam (oil bath for feet)
This treatment is the same as above but you need a plastic container or tub of the size of your feet. The oil should be enough so that your feet can dip in it up to your ankles. Keep your feet for half an hour in the oil. After taking out from the oil, give them a wet and hot treatment for about fifteen minutes with towels dipped in hot water and squeezed.

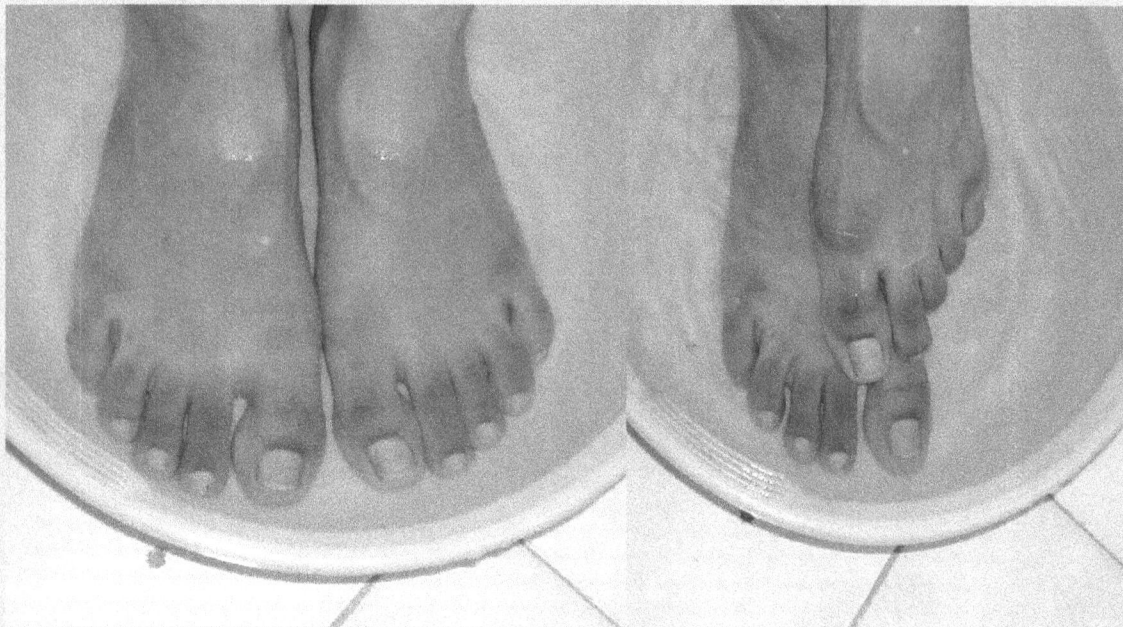

Udram snanam (oil bath for abdomen) Lie down and pour about 30 ml (two table spoons) of warm sesame oil on your navel with the help of a pipette. Soon it will spread around. Spread the already poured oil with your hands everywhere on the abdomen. Repeat this treatment three times. Your whole abdomen will be drenched completely. Give hot treatment as described above with wet and hot towels. Rest for a while after the treatment.

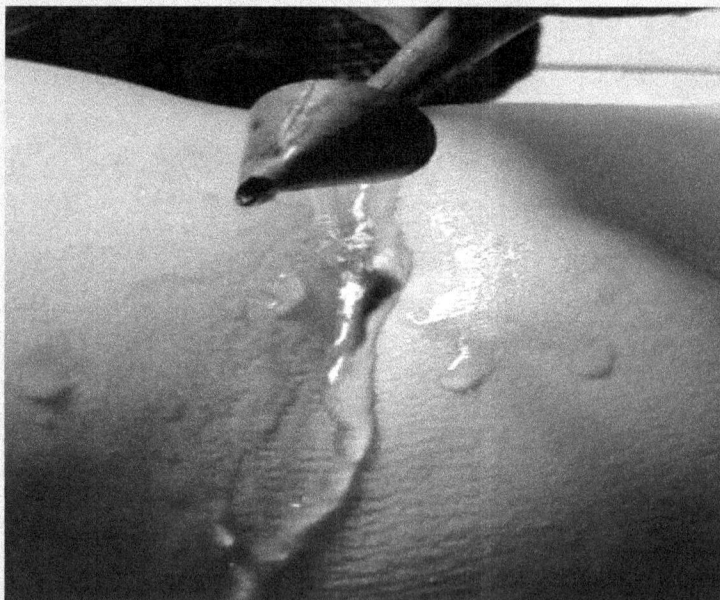

Anointing for balancing the body fire

Pitta imbalance may give you a feeling of burning in the whole body or in certain specific parts of the body. Some people complain of a burning sensation in hands and feet while some others have it on the forehead. The other symptoms of pitta imbalance are excessive sweat and bad smell from the body.

All these symptoms are unpleasant for you and they also make you unattractive for others. Besides taking nutritional and other measures for pitta equilibrium, external anointing will help you immediately and will make your body soft and pleasant smelling.

Anointing with sandalwood paste: Make paste from a peace of sandalwood or from sandalwood powder (see the details of preparations in the eighth chapter of the book). Apply a thin layer of this paste all over your body or only at parts which have burning sensation. Apply by rubbing properly so that your skin assimilates the paste. In case of excessive sweating, it is advisable to put the paste almost everywhere on the body. Leave the anointing for at least an hour and wash it off gradually by rubbing gently.

Anointing with mud: Very fine yellow earth is used for this purpose. It is also called healing earth (multani mitti in Hindi). Make a thin paste with water. Add approximately 4 to 5 times water of the volume of mud. Do the anointing all over your body and leave for about an hour. Wash the mud off by gentle rubbing.

Anointing with fine sand: Like the yellow mud, sand is also cold in nature. Sand is also strength promoting for the bones. It also will make you get rid of small skin irritants or rash. But you need to have very fine sand for this purpose. Smear gently the wet sand on all over your body. Keep rubbing softly for about 15 minutes. Wash it off after about half an hour.

Special padasnanam (foot bath) and padalepa (feet anointing) for smelly feet or feet with fungus

Some people sweat excessively on their feet which smell bad when they wear socks and shoes. Their feet have excessive heat or pitta imbalance. The problem is not limited only to sweating as humidity gives rise to fungus on the toes. To cure this problem, do the mud anointing and sandalwood anointing as described above. Besides taking these measures to create pitta equilibrium, do the following treatment with a decoction of black tea.

Tea footbath and anointing

Boil 3 to 4 litres of water and put two tablespoon of black tea in it. Take the small leaf tea which is technically called the tea dust. English Breakfast tea, PG tea or Brook Bond Red Label tea will serve this purpose. Cover the pot and let the tea cook for about 5 minutes on low fire. Let it lie like this until the temperature lowers down for the footbath. Filter the tea and put it in a plastic tub. Sit down comfortably and dip your feet in it. Keep your feet in it for about 15 minutes. If the decoction cools down, add some hot water in it. Wipe the feet after footbath and put on a clean pair of socks.

You can also make an anointing with tea instead of footbath. Boil about 100 ml of water and add a tablespoon of tealeaves. Let it cook for a few minutes covered. Let it lie like this for few more minutes and filter it. Add about 50 ml of more water in the left over of the tea and boil again for few minutes. Filter this also in the previous decoction. Add about a tablespoon of *besin* (chickpea flour) into this decoction and mix properly to make a paste. If it is too thin for anointing, add a little more *besin*. Smear this paste all over your feet and also between your toes. Leave it like this until it gets completely dry. Rub the dried paste off or wash with warm water.

To feel upbeat with a pressure massage

Pressure massage is specially recommended for persons of kapha prakriti and more so to treat the kapha vikriti. If you feel that you have a droopy appearance and you find yourself lacking all initiative, a pressure massage will do you good immediately. Given below is the method to do pressure massage on your own.

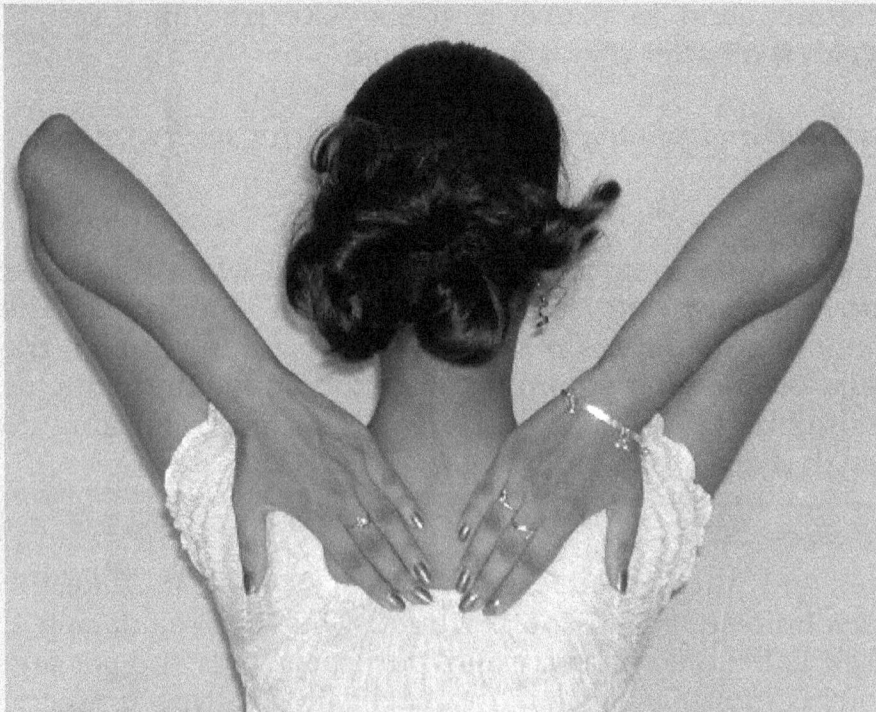

Self- pressure massage
In case of kapha vikriti, you may not take an initiative to go and get a massage in a salon or make another arrangement to get yourself a pressure massage. Help-yourself at home with the following simple methods.

Upper back and neck: Lift both your arms and take your hands behind the upper part of your back in such a way that your palms are facing your back. Start clapping your hands on your back in a rhythmical manner on your neck and upper part of the back. Do not clap gently but apply appropriate pressure. With your hands in this position, you cannot apply excessive pressure. Thus, apply the maximum pressure you can and still you will not hurt yourself.

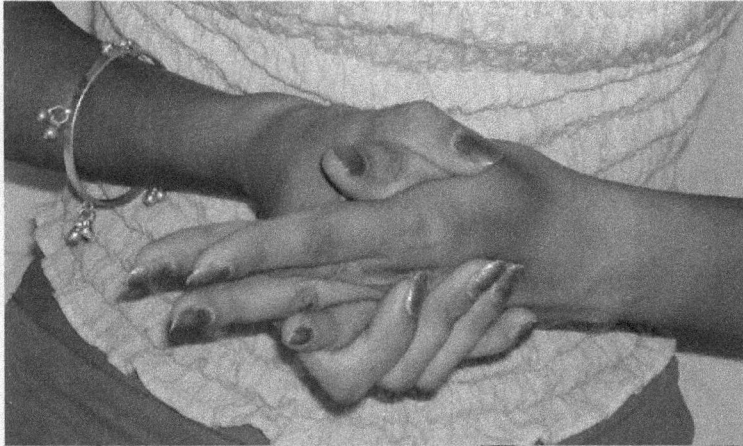

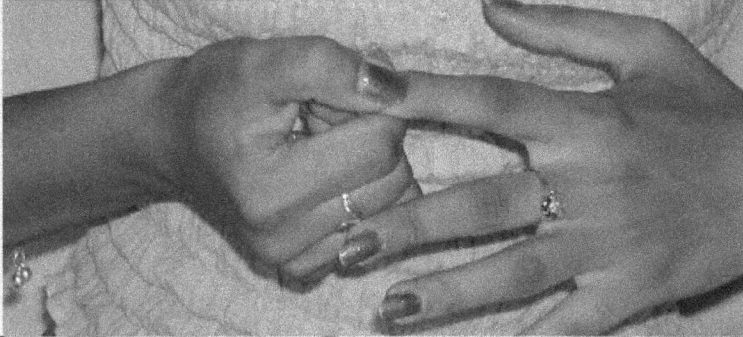

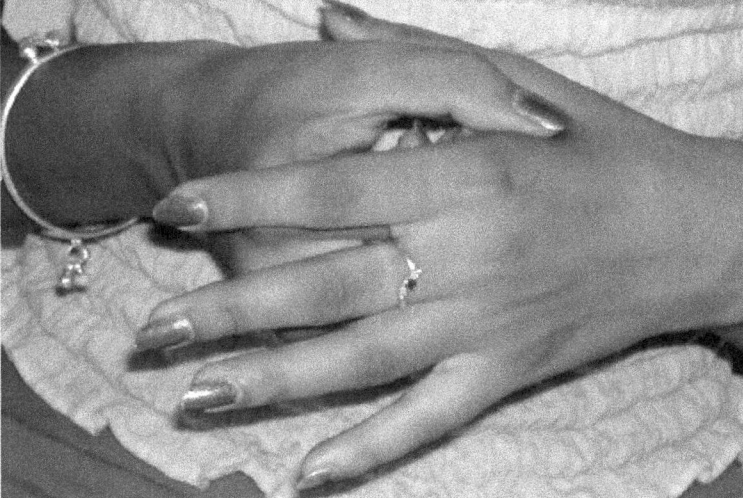

Hands and feet: The above practice will take your drowsy feeling away and will prepare you to do pressure massage on your own in other parts of the body. If you do not have time to do the whole body massage, do at least your hands and feet with pressure on certain specific points to energise yourself.

Start pressing your left hand with your right hand from the tip of your fingers to the wrist. Apply good and well-distributed pressure and keep rotating your left hand so that it gets pressed everywhere. Now pay attention to the individual parts of the hand. Press all your fingers very tightly.

The next step is to take the tip of each finger and press it from all sides. Come down to the place between your fingers and press these from both the sides. Particularly important is the place between the index finger and thumb where the pressure points for the neck regions and throat are lying.

Those of you with some stiffness in neck or pain in throat will have pain in these pressure points.

Press the palm with force and from all sides and end the massage by twisting the hand to the left and to the right to invigorate the wrist. Do your right hand with the left in a similar manner.

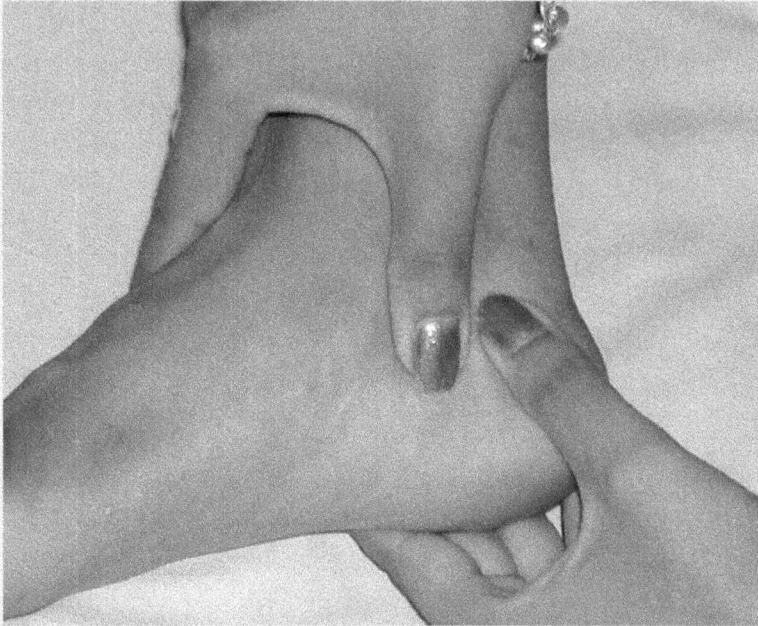

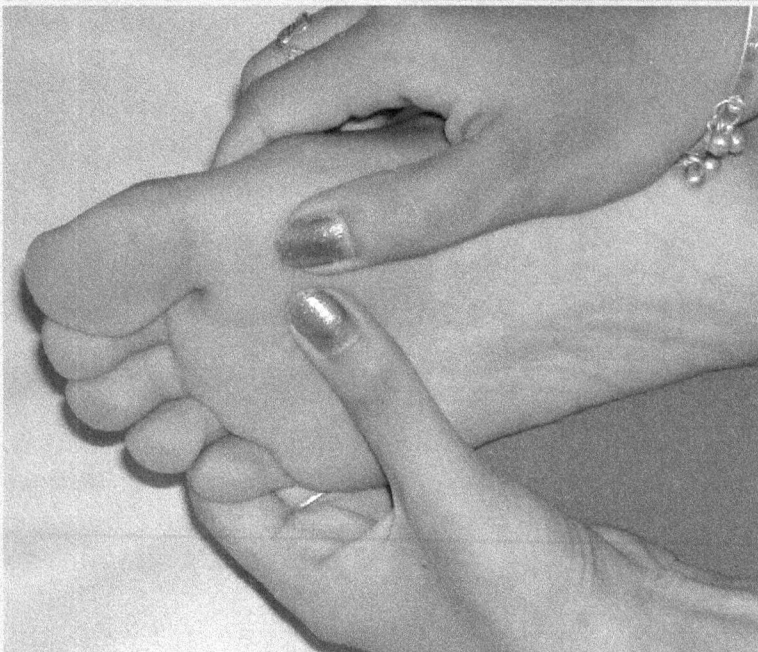

Sit down and hold your left foot in both your hands. Press it from all sides up to the ankle several times. Press the individual fingers and toe, their tips and the space between the fingers as you did for the hand massage. Apply pressure on the toe and the part below it several times. These are important as the pressure points for nerves and brain lie here. With both your thumbs, apply pressure on various parts of the sole, specially the upper part. Similarly, apply pressure to the sides of the feet. Continue applying pressure in the similar manner on the ankle and end the massage by twisting the foot from the ankle.

Arms and legs: Along with hands and feet, you can also extend the pressing massage to your arms and legs. It is easier to press your legs on your own than arms. You cannot apply so much pressure with one hand on your arm.

5
Nutrition and its effect on Health and Beauty

The rational basis of Ayurveda is that the whole cosmos works on the same principle. The five elements make the world of form, colour and smell and that also includes human body. In order to organise all the biological and mental functions of the body, the five elements take the form of three dosha or the three principal energies– vata, pitta and kapha. Obviously these energies need to be replenished and that is done through breathing and nourishment. Nourishment or *ahara* is defined in Ayurveda as all that we eat, drink, lick or devour. All what we take in through our mouth, skin, nose etc. and is assimilated in our body has some effect on the totality of our system. If we get an oil massage, it is also nourishment and our food is also nourishment. Inhalation of etheric oils, smoke of tobacco and pollution, pesticides and the chemicals used for preservation– all these are assimilated in the body. They have their good or bad effects because all that goes inside us affects the three doshas in one way or the other.

Rasa and the five elements

Just as the body is made of five elements, so is the nourishment. The food we eat has diverse tastes, called rasa in Ayurveda and there are six principal rasas. The commonsensical use of the word taste is to define what the tongue experiences and recognizes as sweet, sour, bitter, and so on. However, the term rasa is used in the sense of the total affect that particular taste has on the body.

Let us see why a rasa affects our entire system. Each rasa has two cosmic elements in it. Sweet is constituted of earth and water and bitter is constituted of ether and air. Sour has fire element along with water, saline has fire element along with earth and pungent has fire element along with air. The sixth rasa is astringent and has a combination of earth and air elements. Thus, to nourish ourselves well, we need to include all the rasas in our daily meals so that we can maintain the balance of the three doshas in our body. When the doshas are disturbed and are imbalanced, we can play with the proportions of the diverse tastes in our food to create equilibrium. Thus, besides sustaining the body functions by replenishing the three doshas, food has therapeutic functions when used with wisdom. On the contrary, if discretion is not used, food can be the cause of many health problems. Obesity, diabetes, indigestion, constipation, sleep-disturbances and there are hundreds of other problems caused due to lack of wisdom about what we devour.

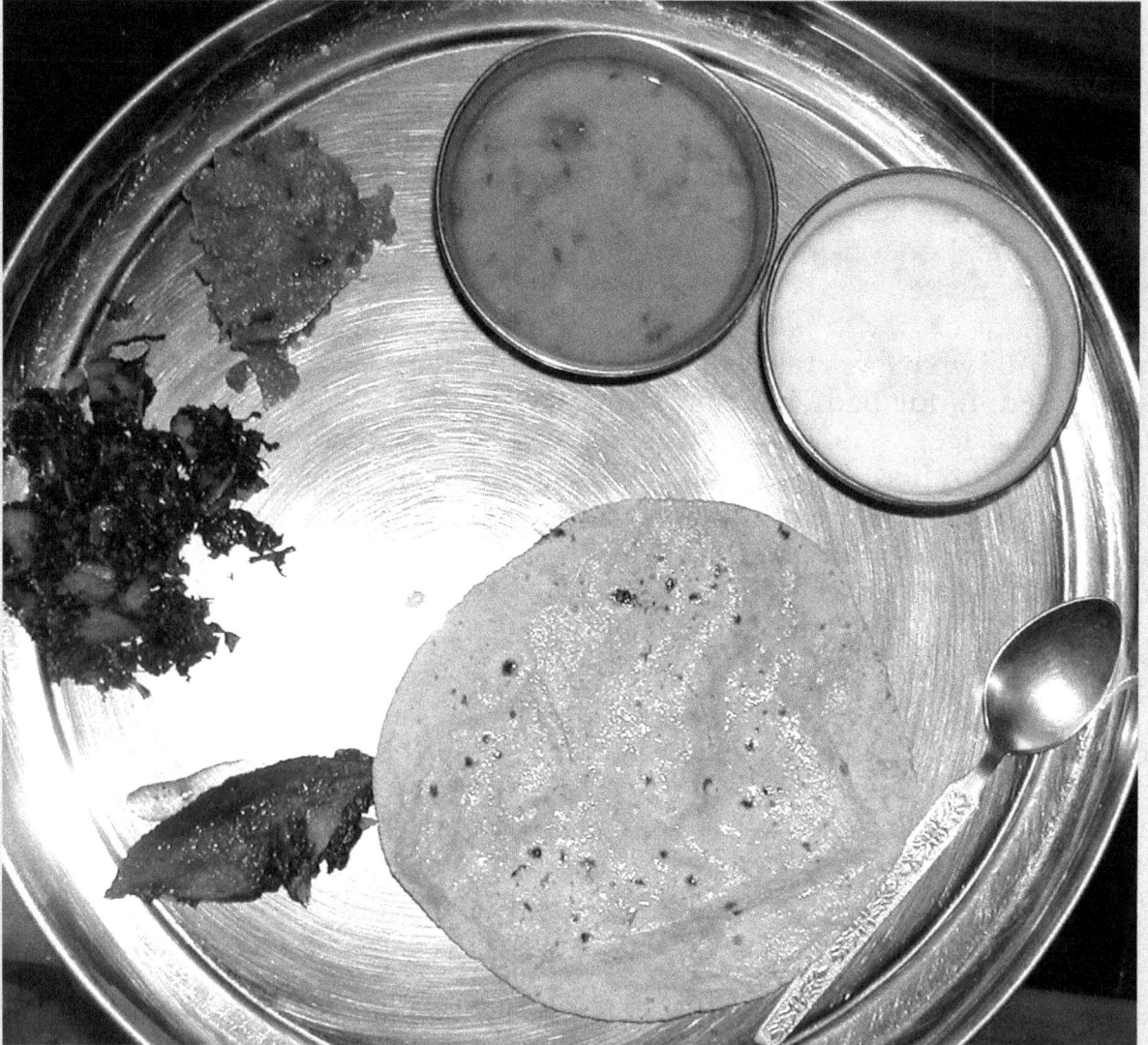

My purpose in this book is not to go into any theoretical details of Ayurvedic nutrition or recipes as I have done that in my other books*. The idea of this chapter in the present book is to make you aware of the affect of nutrition on your appearance and to cure the imbalance that affects your beauty and glamour.

---

1. *Ayurveda for Inner Harmony: Nutrition, Sexual Energy and Healing*, 1992, latest edition available at www.amazon.com
2. *Ayurvedic Food Culture and Recipes*, 2001, latest edition available at www.amazon.com

First of all, I will give you the eight basic precautions you should take. These are integral part of the Ayurvedic food culture. After that, I have listed some principal troubles many people get into due to careless eating habits. I have given the preventions and therapeutic measure in each case.

The eight golden principles of Ayurvedic food Culture

1. Be sure to include all the rasas while **preparing** food. Try to include a variety of ingredients in each meal. Take always warm and fluid food with moderate quantity of fat. Never take preserved foods or those foods which are kept overnight after cooking. Food should be **served** in a beautiful manner to create the congenial and aesthetic atmosphere for its consumption.

2. Never **consume** food under stressful circumstances or under any emotional restraint. If you happen to be in such a state shortly before your meal, wait for a while, do some breathing exercises, wash your face with cold water and then sit comfortably for taking your meal.

3. **Before beginning your meal**, bring your mind to your food, which is the fundamental basis of body's energy. Look at your food and make a wish that the five elements of the food may provide you with equilibrium, vigour and good health. Say a little prayer or take some deep breaths.

4. The food should be **eaten neither too slow nor too fast.** You should not speak with food in the mouth.

5. Ayurveda recommends **drinking** only one hour after the food. If required to drink along with food, one may consume liquid in small quantities. Ayurveda recommends drinking only very good quality of wine or beer in a small quantity with food. Juices and milk should not be taken with food. Water is highly recommended but one hour after the meal. Food should be fluid and should include some soup or something similar.

6. Never eat anything **before the previous meal is completely digested.** According to Ayurveda, it is poisonous for the body if one eats when the body is still in the process of digesting the previous meal. Do not eat anything four hours after having eaten something. For your stomach, a little thing like a piece of chocolate or a fruit is also food to be worked upon and digested. Thus, strictly do not eat anything between meals. If due to

some heavy food, you are not hungry for the next meal even after 5 or 6 hours, then avoid taking a meal or take something very light like a soup.

7. Many people in the world make themselves sick by eating too much. According to Ayurveda, you should always eat that much quantity, which fills the **stomach two third and not completely full**. It means, eat to the limit when you feel comfortably satisfied and not so full that you cannot eat any more. Logic of this is that the three doshas also require place in the stomach for the digestion of the food. If the stomach is made full to its utmost capacity, during digestion, the humours are pushed out and give rise to vitiation causing thereby various digestive troubles. This may also give rise to *amadosha*. Amadosha is the partial digestion of the food and undigested food remains in the stomach and intestines, ultimately leading to toxicity in the whole body. For the well-being of the body and for avoiding serious ailments related to digestion, it is absolutely essential to have discipline about the quantity of food you consume.

8. Never take a shower or bath immediately after eating. Wait at least two hours, preferably three hours. In any case, it is better to have shower or bath before eating. Also avoid any form of vigorous exercise after food. All these vitiate vata. Going for a slow walks after dinner is highly recommended.

Make and effort to follow the above principles and you will get a feeling of a general well being. It is quite possible that some of your nagging troubles like heaviness, fatigue, constipation, acidity are cured and your complexion is better. Go through the problems given below and take precautions for your specific case.

Problems in appearance related to food

Consuming imbalanced food and not abiding by the eight golden principles of Ayurvedic nutrition have a bad effect on our health and appearance. There are problems of health that you cannot perceive until there are symptoms of a disorder like stomach ache or a bad taste in mouth. But the changes in outward appearance are well perceivable and can inspire you to change your food habit. Keeping this in mind, I have specifically listed below the problems of nutrition related to appearance and solutions are given thereafter.

Problem 1
Weight imbalance

The first and foremost is the problem of over-weight that troubles a large number of people around the world. Under-weight is also a problem in some cases, especially in children. I am not taking into account any weight imbalance due to ailments. Largely people put on weight due to eating in excess and too many fatty, salty and sweet products and their activities are not in proportion to the food they eat. There are others who eat a lot but still do not have the appropriate weight. There is a third category that has generally loss of appetite and due to that they eat little and are under-weight.

Solutions

Weight loss: Over-weight is an enormous problem in the world and for treating this it, refer to my book on this theme*. I will give you some very basic instructions here which are related to your nutrition so that you do not get a sickly appearance and wrinkles in the process of losing weight.

- Do not follow fat free diets or the chemical drugs that throw out in your excreta all the fat you consume. Your body needs fat and without it, you will get vata imbalance. Reduce the quantity of fat and increase your physical activities. But if you stop the intake of fat, you will acquire a dull complexion with rough skin due to vata imbalance.
- Go on a rigorous mission to lose weight. Reduce the intake of fat, sugar and salt. Increase the intake of vegetables and fruits. Take papaya almost everyday. Avoid bananas. Eat vegetarian food with spices like cumin, pepper, ginger, fenugreek, coriander, etc. (see my above-referred book for more details). Avoid eating grains, as they are bulk promoting. Cook with very little oil and from time to time with ghee. Use non-stick pans so that you can prepare low-fat food.
- Avoid buying pre-prepared things which have already salt or sugar. Prepare everything fresh and from basic ingredients. Eat warm and fluid food and not dry and cold.
- Follow all the eight golden principles of Ayurvedic food culture.

Gaining weight: If you eat a lot and still stay thin, your pitta energy is vitiated. You need medical help. The problem can be of diverse sort. If the following nutritional and self-help measures do not help, consult a physician.

---

* *Losing Weight with Yoga and Ayurveda*, latest edition available at www.amazon.com

- In case you have frequent and excessive stool, drink decoction of fennel. Fennel loses its medicinal qualities if boiled to make decoction. Method of making cold decoction is called *phant* in Ayurveda. Take two teaspoon of fennel and pour 1L hot water on it. Let it lie overnight and next day drink this water during the day whenever you are thirsty. You can either filter it or just chew the fennel seed along with your drink. If you do not like to drink at room temperature, you can warm it but do not heat it.
- Increase the use of fennel and coriander as a spice in your meals. Take them in equal quantity and grind them. I have named it as Mixture C or the Cooling Mixture in my food book. Use this spice mixture in your food preparations.
- Take nutmeg and mace as spice in your soups and other dishes.
- Eat bulk-promoting foods like grain preparations. Maize (called corn in North America) and chickpea flour (*besan*) are specially recommended.
- Ghee and other products from milk are bulk promoting but take them according to your digestive capacity.
- In the process of gaining weight, do not over-eat. Follow all the golden rules given above. If you eat too frequently and too much, you will spoil your system even more.
- To get a sound sleep, drink hot milk with saffron and candy sugar before going to bed. Milk is sleep-inducing. Sleep is bulk promoting.
- Include bananas and avocados in your food.

Loss of appetite: Here are some instructions to increase appetite.

- Enhance the use of fresh ginger in your food. Eat fresh ginger slices with rock salt and lemon juice on them half an hour before meals. Since children will not like to eat ginger like this, give them fresh ginger juice in water along with candy sugar and lemon juice before meals.
- Ajwain (*Trachyspermum ammi*) is common Indian spice also available at Indian stores abroad. It is something like thyme but ajwain seeds are used. Use this in your soups and vegetables for promoting appetite. Take half teaspoon of ajwain with a little lemon juice and a pinch of rock salt to cure indigestion and promote appetite.
- Use pepper, long pepper (peepal), cumin and dill seeds in your food preparations.

Problem 2
Dull and rough complexion

As I have already stated above, a dull and rough complexion is due to vata imbalance. Those who eat cold and dry food (biscuits, bread and other foods with long shelf-life, dried meats, etc.), preserved, hard and rough foods (e.g. frozen pizzas warmed up in microwave oven) usually get dull and rough complexion. Mostly these persons also have problems of constipation or partial evacuation.

Solutions
- Change your food habits and get used to cooking simple but fresh food each time.
- Take preparations with rice, semolina, pasta and whole-wheat flour.
- Consume plenty of fresh vegetables and fruits. Eat fruit salads with papaya, banana and other fruits.
- Make sure that you have a soup for dinner everyday.
- Make a spice mixture with fennel, cumin, coriander, mustard seeds, kalonji, dill seeds and fenugreek in equal quantity. This mixture is not ground. Use this spice mixture in your food preparations. Shake the bottle each time before use so that you get all the ingredients in your spoon full of spices.

Problem 3
Excessive sweating and Body smell
This happens due to the disturbance of your pitta energy.

Solutions
- Take cold milk, wheat and rice preparations. Avoid preparations of soya beans.
- Spinach, cabbage, green beans, bitter gourd (karela), endives, aubergine, cucumber, sweet paprika, beetroot and asparagus are some of the cooling vegetables. Avoid cress, potatoes, cauliflower and tomatoes. Moong beans, carrots and turnips are recommended.
- Sweet fruits like banana, pear, sweet grapes, melons should be taken frequently. Sour fruits and other sour foods should be avoided.
- Herbs and spices like coriander, fennel, clove, anise and liquorice should be used frequently.
- Avoid eating strong smelling foods all together. Do not eat garlic, onions, fenugreek, kalonji and mustard until your problem is gone. Besides their smell, these spices are also hot in their Ayurvedic nature and they make you sweat.
- Use ghee instead of oils for cooking.
- If you are a meat eater, eat only fish, mutton and chicken until you are cured.

- Take bitter vegetables or other bitter substances.

Problem 4
Dull appearance and a 'drag personality'

This problem comes due to kapha imbalance. One suffers from the problem of lassitude and looks and feels dull.

Solutions
- Enhance the use of spices like ginger, garlic, cumin, pepper, big cardamom, dill seeds, kalonji, and fenugreek in your meals.
- Reduce the intake of sweet and oily foodstuffs.
- Take sour fruits like grapefruit, orange, pineapple, kiwi, plumbs and peaches.
- Avoid milk, ghee and butter. Instead take oil, yoghurt and cheese but in small quantity.
- Avoid wheat, rice and maize preparations. Include preparations from soya beans in your menu.

Problem 5
Pimples, Herpes, blisters in mouth and other skin eruptions

These problems arise due to pitta imbalance and mala (impurities and toxin) in the blood.

Solution
You will need to follow a multiple programme to get rid of these problems. Take all the precautions described above in problem number 3. Take bitter teas and some blood purifying preparations described on page 65. In case these problems persist, you need to purify yourself with panchakarma practices.

6

Yoga and Yogic Dance to Enhance Health and Charm

Flexibility of the body and a proper distribution of energy in the body are primary to good health and attractive appearance. The classical dancers of diverse Indian dances learn yoga from their childhood and that enables them to command each movement and each muscle of their body. Indian classical dances are not merely the bodily movements but a total harmony of body, mind and soul. I do not have a scientific data, but my general observation reveals that the classical dancers live long and healthy lives. Whatever is your age, you can make your body flexible with gradual effort through yogic movements. I have done research on movements of yoga and nritya (the Indian classical dances) and have developed a slow motion yogic nritya, which can be used to enhance your beauty, charm and health. I have given four different programmes to be done in four steps to make your body gradually flexible before you begin yogic dance.

Energy is distributed in the body through energy channels called srotas in Ayurveda. Due to inactivity or less activity, the srotas get closed and energy distribution system of the body is disturbed. Our body has possibilities for many diverse movements and if we do not use these possibilities, gradually we lose our flexibility. It is not enough to do some walking, jogging or other work with movements to keep body flexible. Yogabhyasa (yogic exercises) and yogasanas (yogic postures) open the energy channels, exercise the internal organisms of the body and give you a glowing complexion. It is a very vast subject and I have written a lot on this theme in all my books. However, in the present contexts, I will give certain specific exercises for getting a good complexion and flexibility. I strongly recommend doing a set of 12 yogic exercises called Surya Pranam (salutation to the Sun), 12 times a day after drinking hot water in the morning and relieving yourself. I have described these in my other books. However, beginners need to learn simpler yogic exercises before learning Surya Pranam.

Yoga programme in four steps

I have made this programme in such a way that your body can become gradually flexible without any excessive strain or muscular tension. Each step contains five yogic exercises (yogabhyasa) or yogic postures (yogasanas). Repeat each exercise or posture 3-5 times. I suggest that to begin with, you do each step every week. By repetition, you will learn to do them well and will be handling your body gently. The second reason to follow this programme in steps is the constraint of time most people complain of. Even if you do not have too much time, you can choose to do one step for 8 to 10 minutes to open up your srotas or energy channels. However, on weekends, you should take time to do all the four steps.

Those of you who are never exposed to yoga may find some familiar movements that you learnt from many other methods of exercise inspired from yoga. Keep in mind that the principal difference between yogabhyasa and other exercises is that the body movement in yoga is very slow and the mind should be concentrated on the movements and postures (asana) you are making.

Breathing during yogasanas: I have already explained earlier in the book about the controlled and conscious breathing in yoga called pranayama and have described some practices in Chapter 3. The following practices are presented in such a way that your breathing gradually orients with your movements. Normally, when you do a movement or make a posture, breathing regulates itself automatically. You should never force yourself to hold your breath with force. Prolong the time of the posture very gradually and you will simultaneously get used to prolonging the breath as well. In some specific postures or exercises where it is needed, I have given the breathing pattern. In others, let the body organise itself.

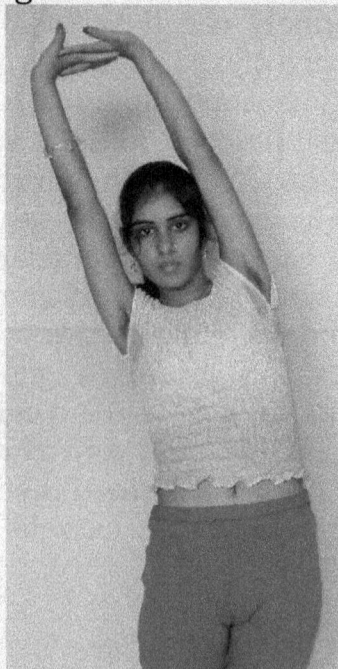

Step I

I give below some very easy set of yogic practices and you can do them with facility even if you are a beginner. All postures or exercise given in this step are done standing.

Yogabhyasa number 1

Stand straight, let yourself loose and raise both your arms. Clasp both your hands together and turn the palms upwards. Make round movements clockwise by moving your waist in circles. Make sure that your head stays within both your arms and your movements are very slow. Concentrate your mind on these rotary movements. Make 3 to 5 movements. Rest for 2-3 breaths and make the same number of movements anticlockwise.

This exercise is energising for abdominal region (stomach and intestines) as well as for neck, shoulders and waist.

Yogabhyasa number 2

Bend forward, clasp both your hands together with the palms facing downwards. Stay like this for a little while and then move on your left side from the waist in such a way that your clasped hands are almost on the side of your left leg. Do the same for the right side.

This exercise energises the lower back, abdomen and arms.

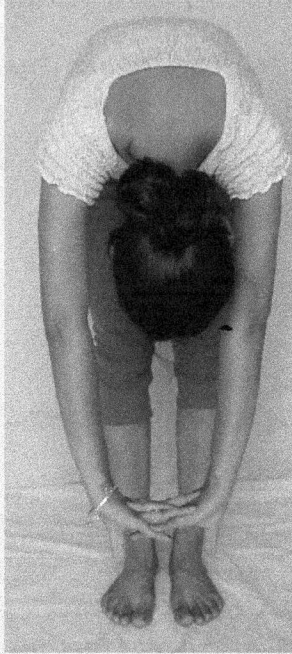

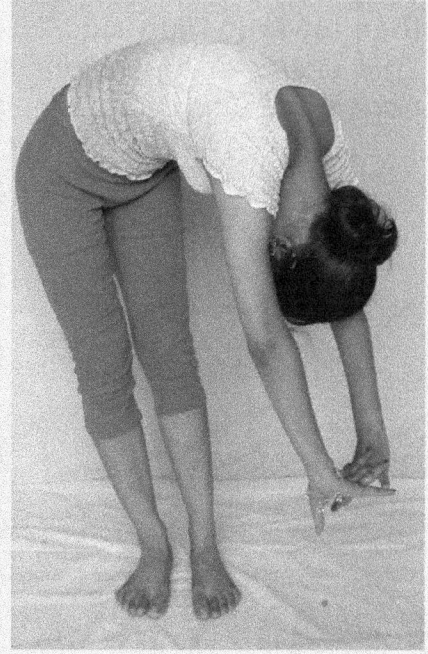

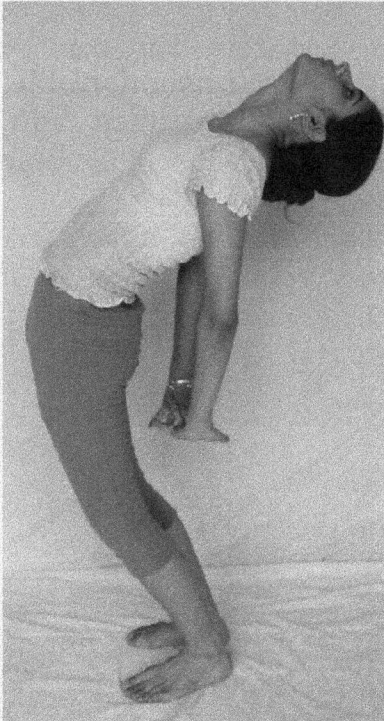

Yogabhyasa number 3

This exercise is nearly the same as number 2 but you are bending backwards with clasped hands. Make the movements on the left and right sides respectively.

This exercise is good for shoulders, neck, chest and respiratory system.

Yogabhyasa number 4

Stand straight and put both your hands at your back and clasp them. Bend forward gradually and keep taking your clasped hands upwards. Stay like this for a while and then curve your waist towards left side. Come back to the original position again and then towards right side.

This exercise is good for shoulders, arms, neck and abdominal muscles.

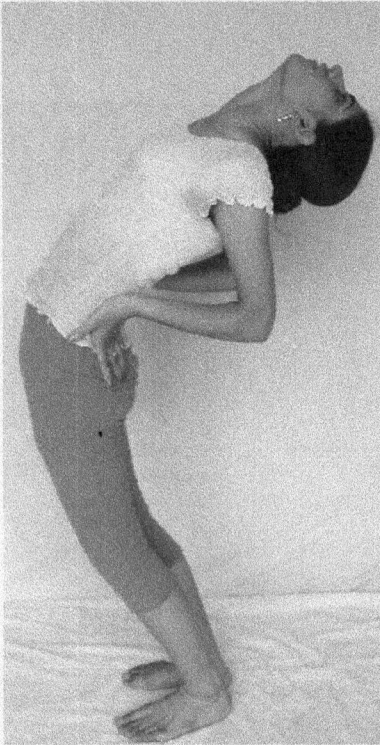

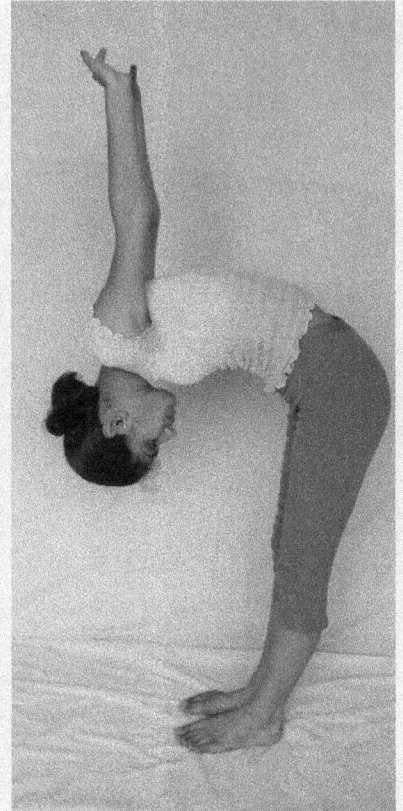

Yogasana number 5

Stand straight and put both your hands on your hips with palms facing inwards. Bend backwards as much as you can without being uncomfortable. Do not get discouraged if you find yourself stiff. Gradually, with constant effort, you will get flexible and will be able to bend more.

This asana makes your backbone flexible, saves you from wrinkles in the neck and from double chin. It opens energy channels of your face muscles. It is very good for the respiratory system.

Step II

This set of yogic practices is done in sitting or half-sitting posture.

Yogasana number 1

Sit down on your heels. Make sure your torso is straight. Put both your hands at your back and hold them together. Bend forwards to rest your head on the floor. Stay in this posture as long as you can comfortably.

This posture enhances the blood flow in your face and exercises your knees and stomach muscles.

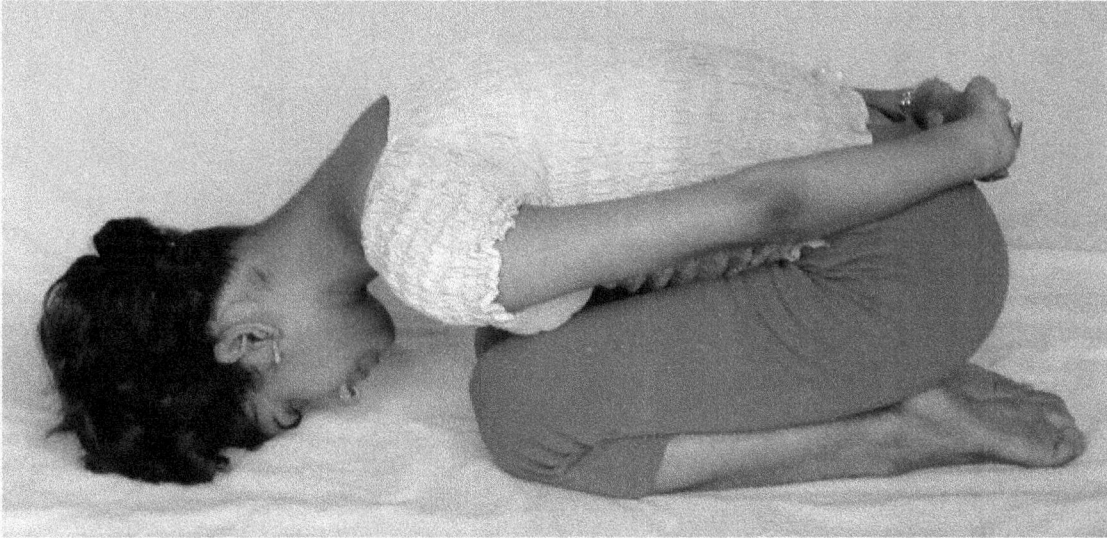

Yogasana number 2

Make the same posture as in number 1 and gradually stretch your clasped hands upwards. Stay in this position as long as you can comfortably and gradually try to increase the duration.

This posture exercises your shoulders and opens srotas in the pectoral region, neck and face. It is a very good posture for getting a glow on your face. It activates your whole body and enhances your memory by energising the brain srotas.

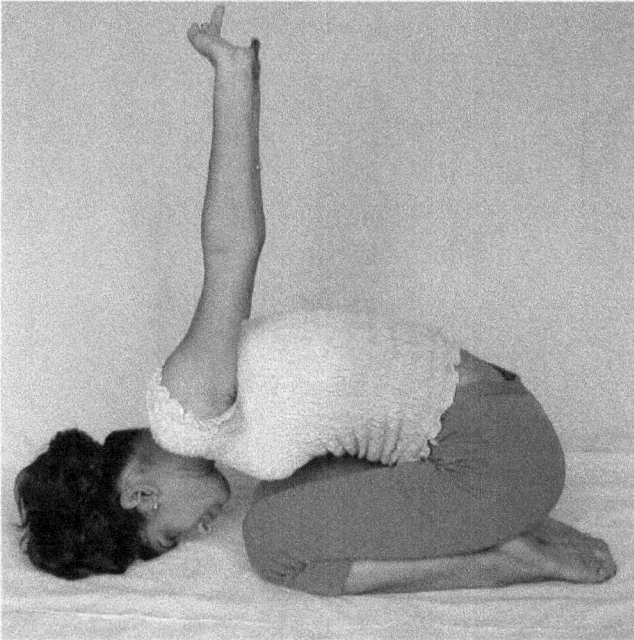

Yogabhyasa number 3

Kneel down and make sure that rest of your body is straight. Walk on your knees and take five steps forward and five steps backwards.

This exercise makes your pelvic and knees joints strong and makes your leg movements flexible.

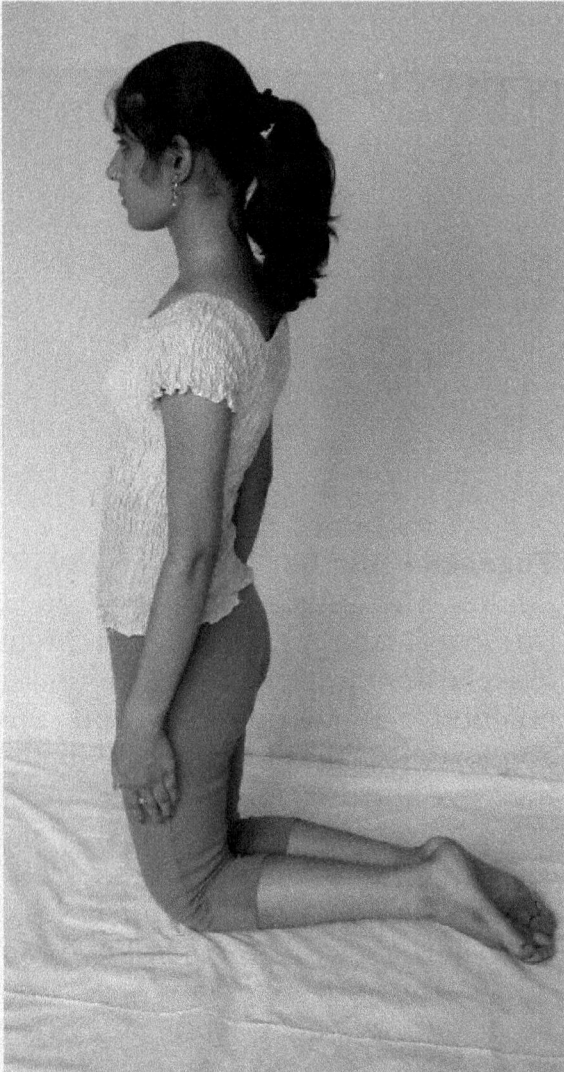

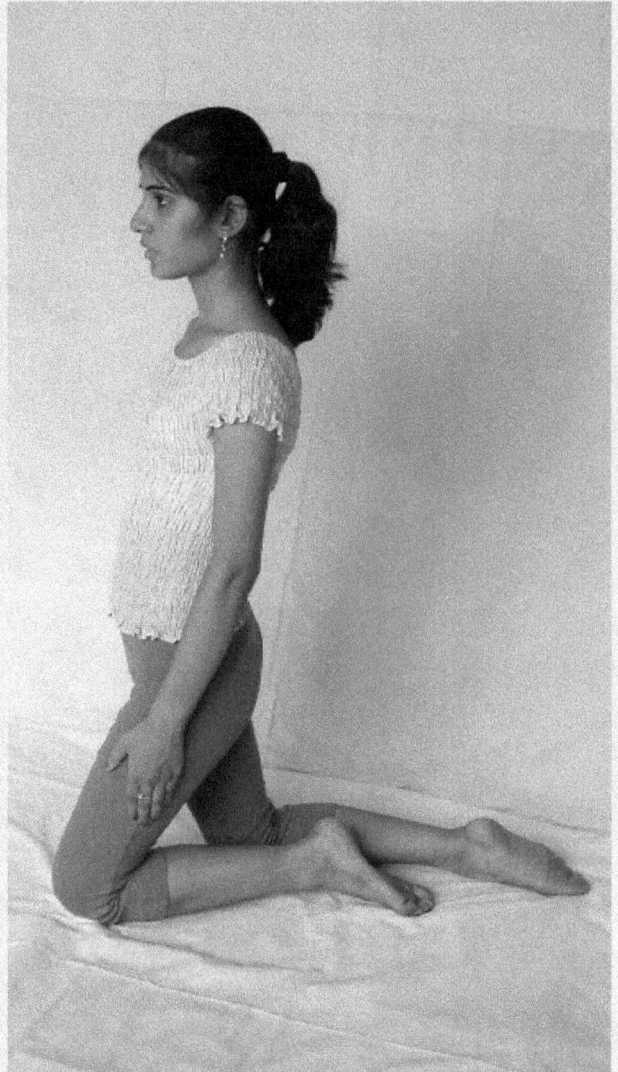

Yogabhyasa number 4
Stand on your knees as above. Put your left foot forward, keep your left hand on your left knee while keeping the right hand straight, parallel to your right thigh. Bring your torso as much forward as you can. Come back to the straight position again. Take a rest of few breaths and repeat the same with your right leg.

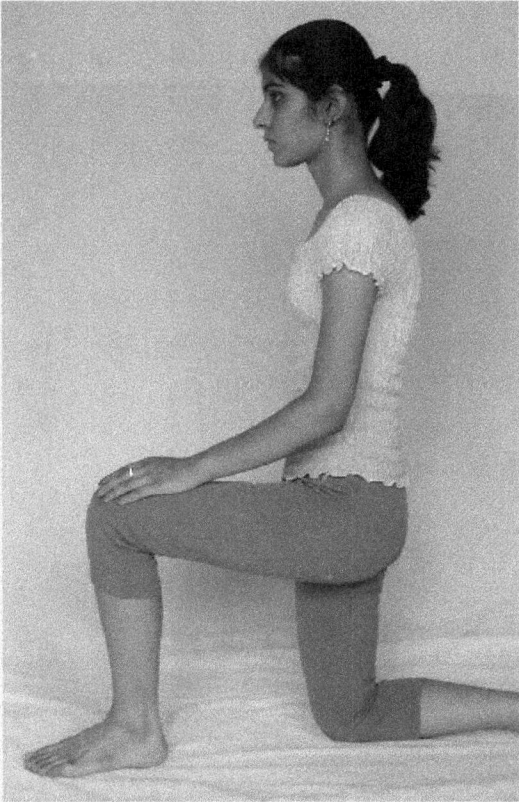

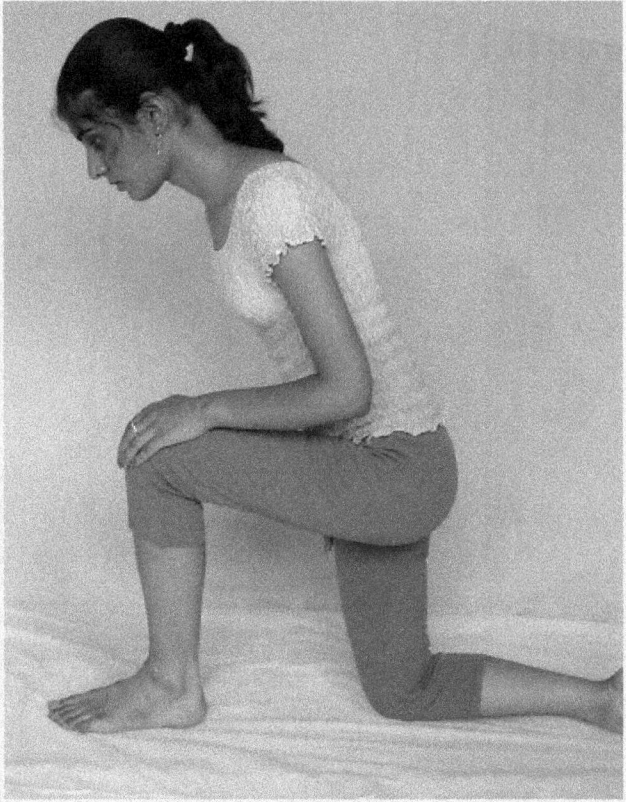

This is a very good exercise for the lower back and pelvic joints. It also open srotas of the internal organs located in the lower part of our body (Kidneys, bladder and sex organs).

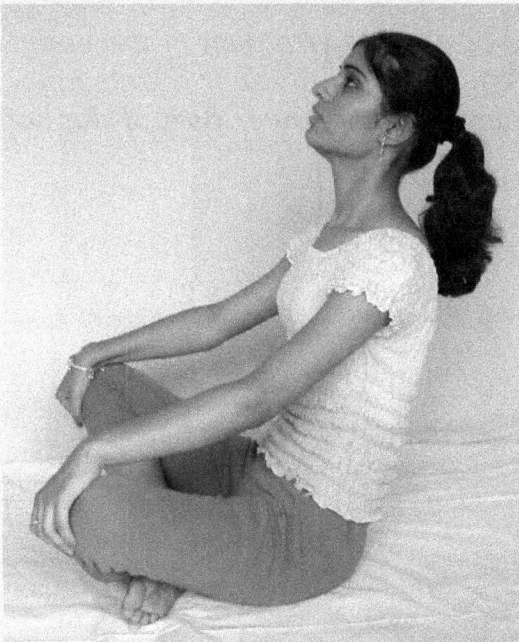

Yogabhyasa number 5

Sit cross-legged and put your hands on your knees. Make forward and backward movements at a very slow pace. Your back should not bend and the movements should be made from the lower back. Go three to four times forward and backward and then bend forward as much as you can. If your body is flexible, you will be able to touch the floor with your forehead. In any case, do not force yourself. You will gain the flexibility gradually.

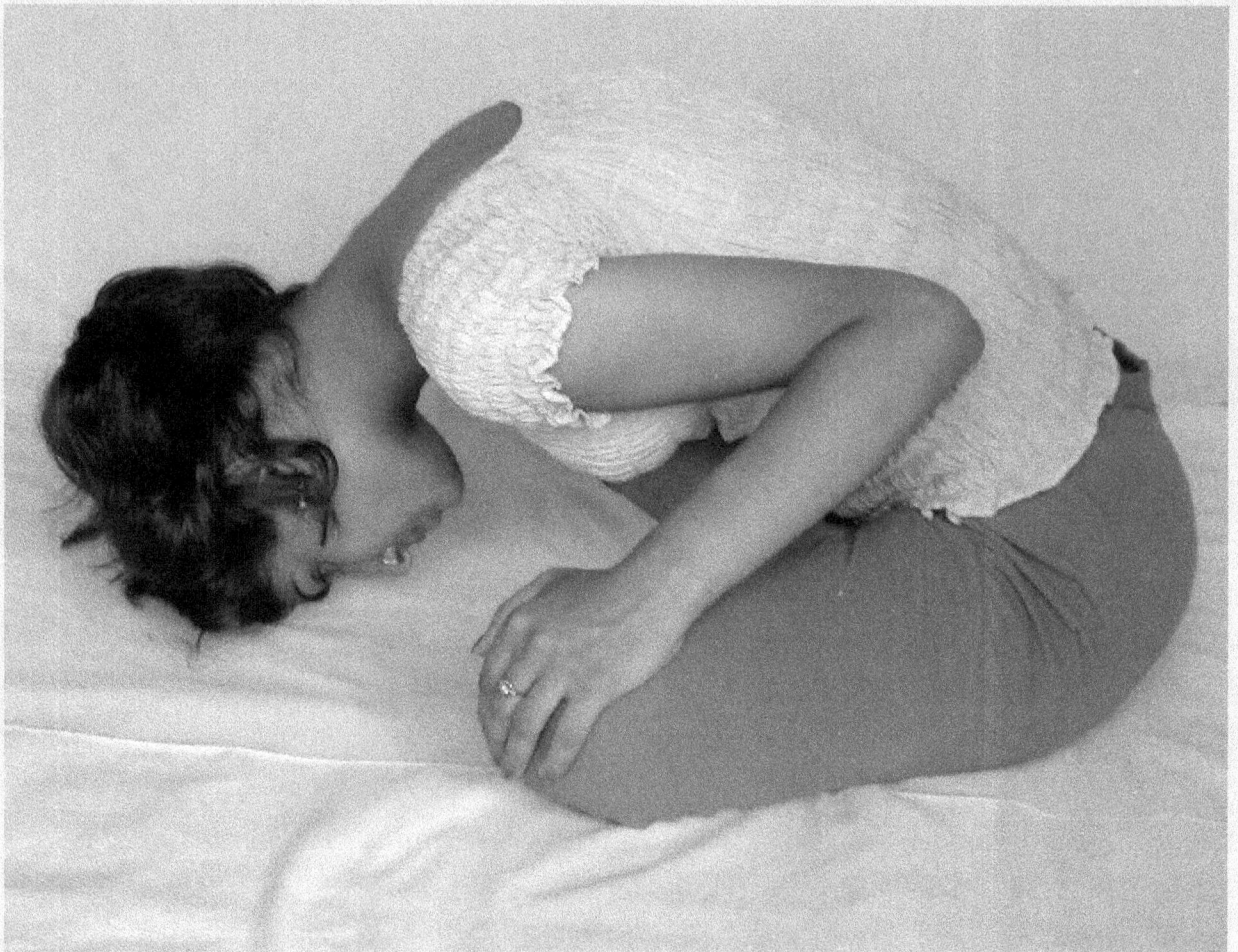

As the above exercise, this exercise also works on the lower region of the body. It provides stability and flexibility to the pelvic region. Both, number 4 and 5 yogic practices help you get the balance of kapha energy as the lower part of the body represents the water and earth elements.

Step III
The yogic practices given in this section are done while laying down.

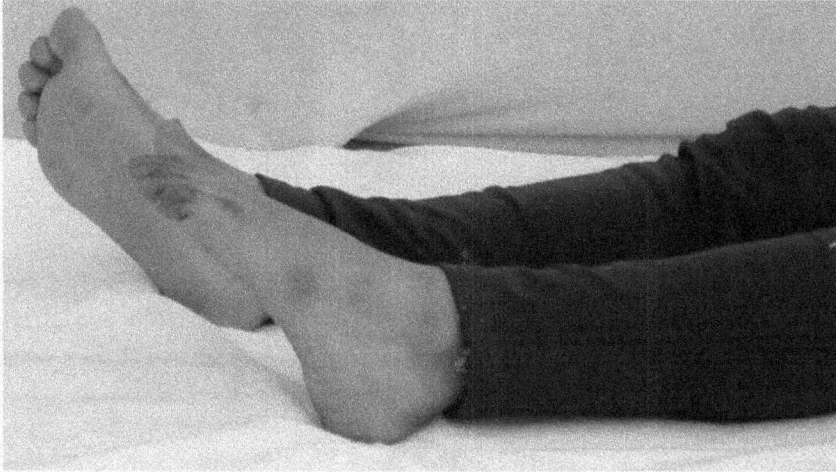

Yogabhyasa number 1
Lie on your back. Let yourself loose. Keep your hands about 30 cm away from your body. Put your feet also about 30 cm apart from each other. Concentrate on your feet and move them clockwise.
The movements should be made very slowly and you should make big circles; as big as the flexibility of your ankle allows you to do. Make sure that rest of your body is completely relaxed. Many people make their hands tense in this process. After about five circles, rest for few breaths and make five anti-clockwise circles.
These exercises not only make your ankle joints flexible but also exercise certain leg muscles on the dorsal parts. In fact, during this exercise, you realise it yourself that you can feel these movements up to your lower back.

Yogasana number 2 and 3
These positions are called Pavanamuktasana (wind release asana). In our abdomen, some wind is trapped from time to time. These asanas are meant for the release of this wind.

Lie down on your back and let yourself completely loose. Fold your left leg so that your knee faces towards your head and your foot is in the air. Put your arms around the knee and clasp your hands together. Simultaneously, lift up your head and pull the knee towards your nose to touch the knee with it. Stay in this posture as long as you can comfortably. Release the knee, straighten your lifted head and make the leg straight in a slow motion. Rest for few breaths and repeat the same with the right leg. Do not feel discouraged if you are unable to touch your knee with your nose. It means some parts of your vertebral column are not flexible enough. Do not force yourself. Try to make this position after a hot bath. Do persistently everyday, taking the knee and the neck a few millimetre closer each day.

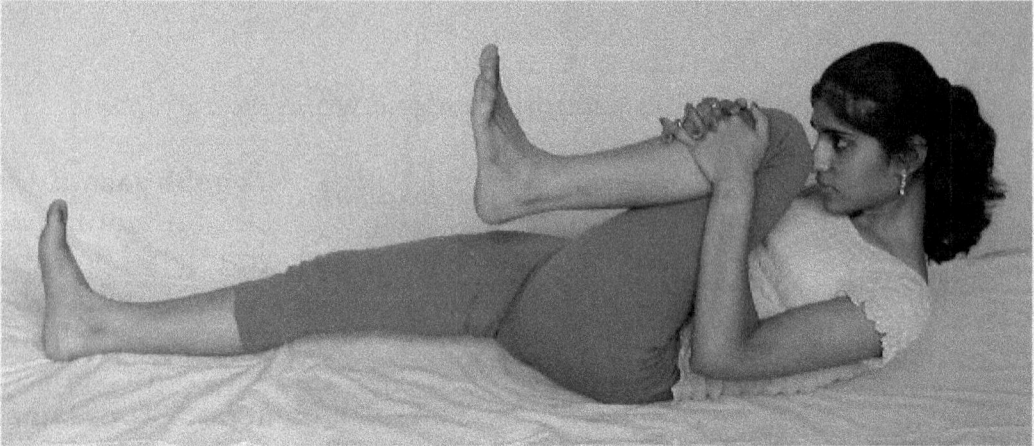

The next asana is done with both the legs together. Put your hands around both your lifted legs and bring your nose in the middle of your knees. Stay in the position as long as you can. As always, try to increase the duration of the asana each time in small gradations.

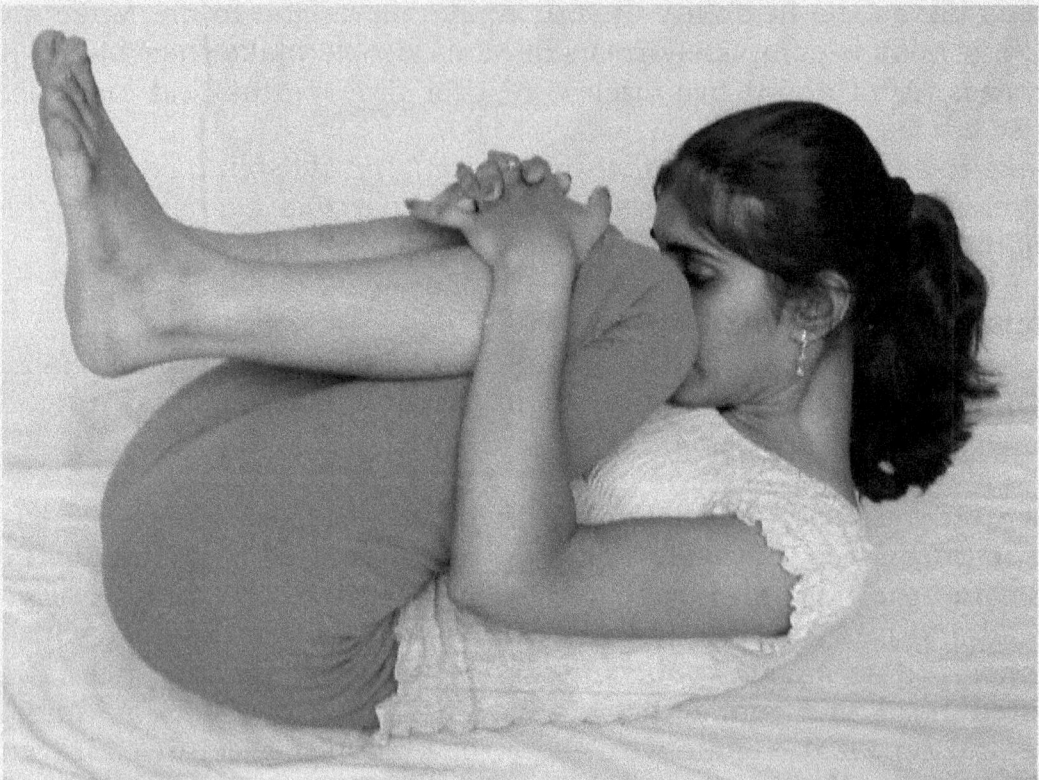

Yogasana number 4

Lie down on your back and completely relax by letting yourself loose. Lift your left leg and put the foot besides the outer part of the right knee. Your sole should be flat on the ground. Stay for a short while in this position and then repeat the same with the right leg.

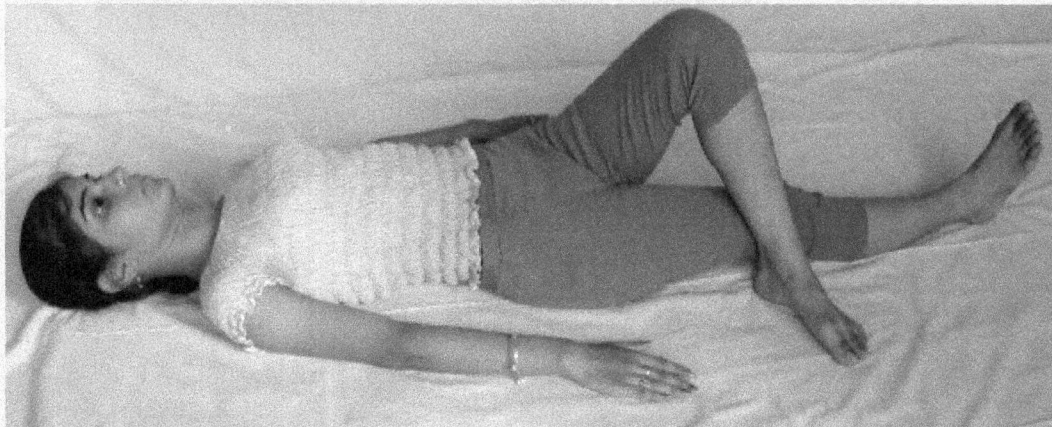

This posture exercises some of those pelvic and abdominal muscles which are not used in day to day activities.

Yogasana number 5

Lie down on your back with arms stretched upwards. Keep lying like this for a short moment until you are completely relaxed. Then start sliding both your arms gradually to bring them parallel to your torso. The arms are not lifted from the ground but are gradually slid making a semi circle with them.
This exercise helps you straighten your shoulder posture and strengthen the shoulder joints.

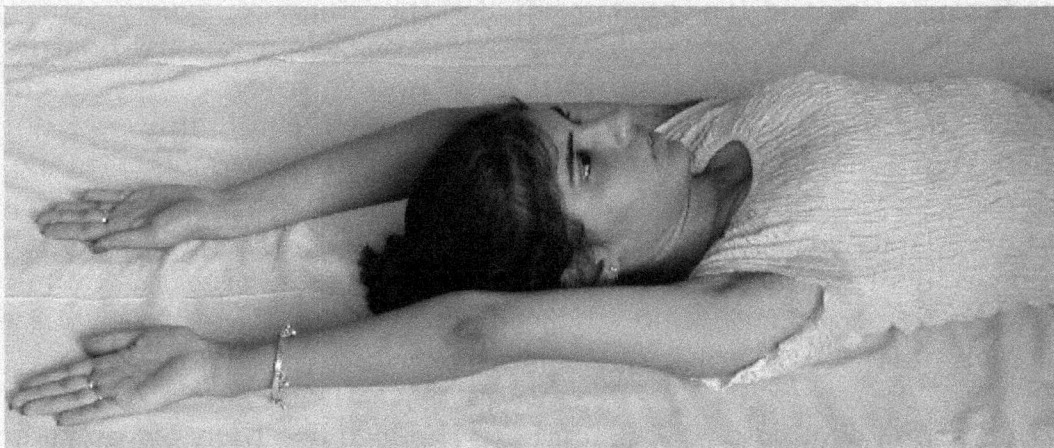

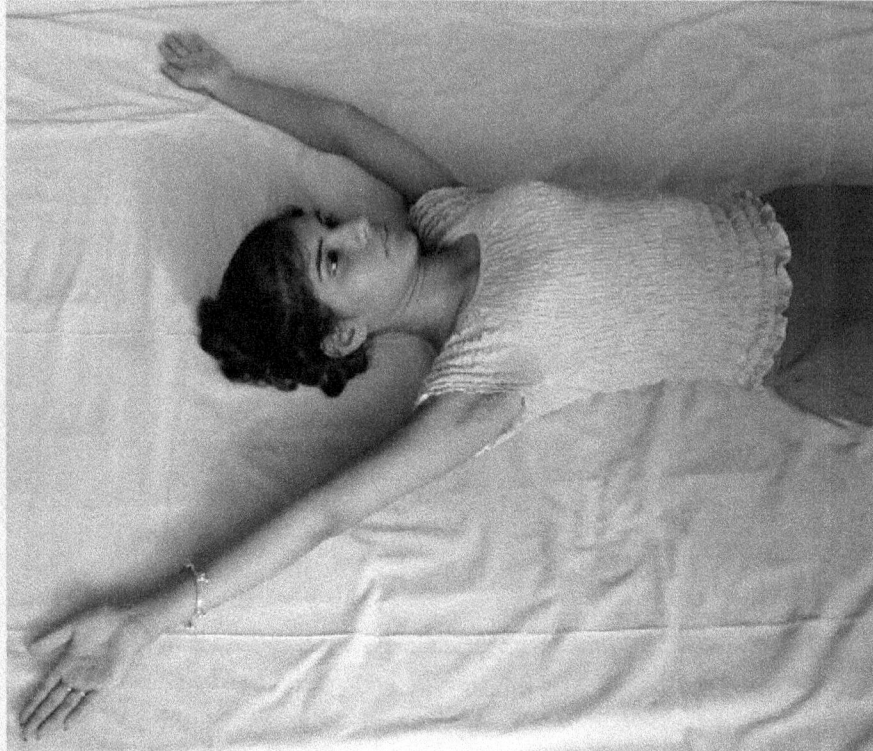

Step IV

You will learn five **advanced asanas** in this section. Therefore it is essential that you do these after you are well versed in above described practices.

Yogasana number 1 and 2

Uttanpadasanas (raised-leg postures): As the name suggests, this asana consists of raising your legs. Lie down on your back in a relaxed posture, with your arms about 30 cm apart from your body and your legs about 30 cm apart from each other. Raise your left leg very slowly while inhaling. Do not bend your knee, your force of lifting should come from your pelvic joint. Inhale in the same rhythm as you are lifting your leg. When you have raised your leg to its maximum capacity, stay in this posture and hold the breath for a moment. Bring down the leg gradually while exhaling. After a brief rest, make this posture with the right leg. Make these asanas about five times with a brief interval each time.

The second asana comprises of raising both the legs together. Lie down on your back and join both your feet. Let yourself loose. Raise both your legs together while inhaling in a similar manner as above. Make sure that your feet stay together all the time. Hold the breath the moment you have raised your legs completely. Bring down your legs slowly while exhaling.

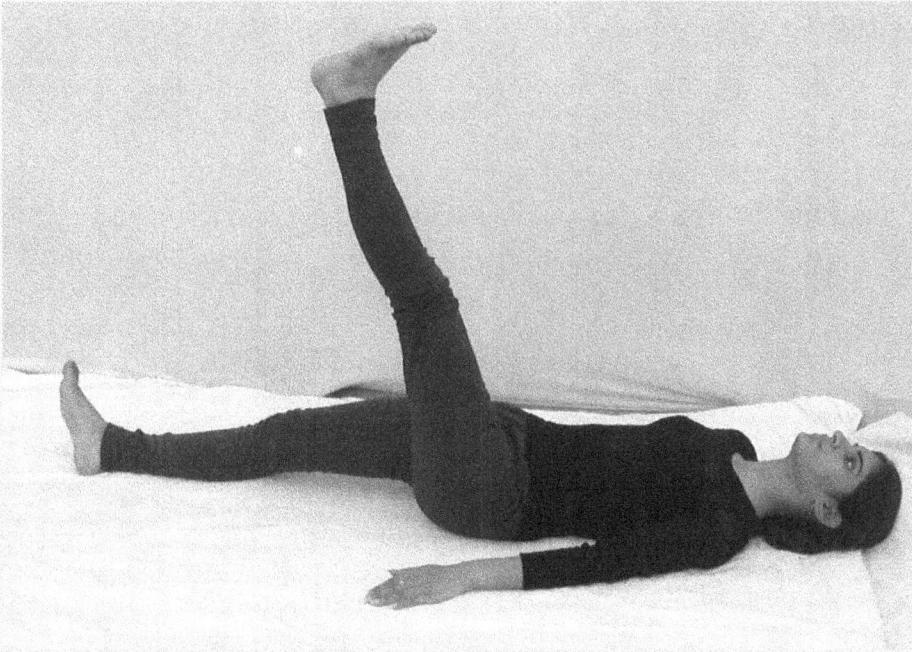

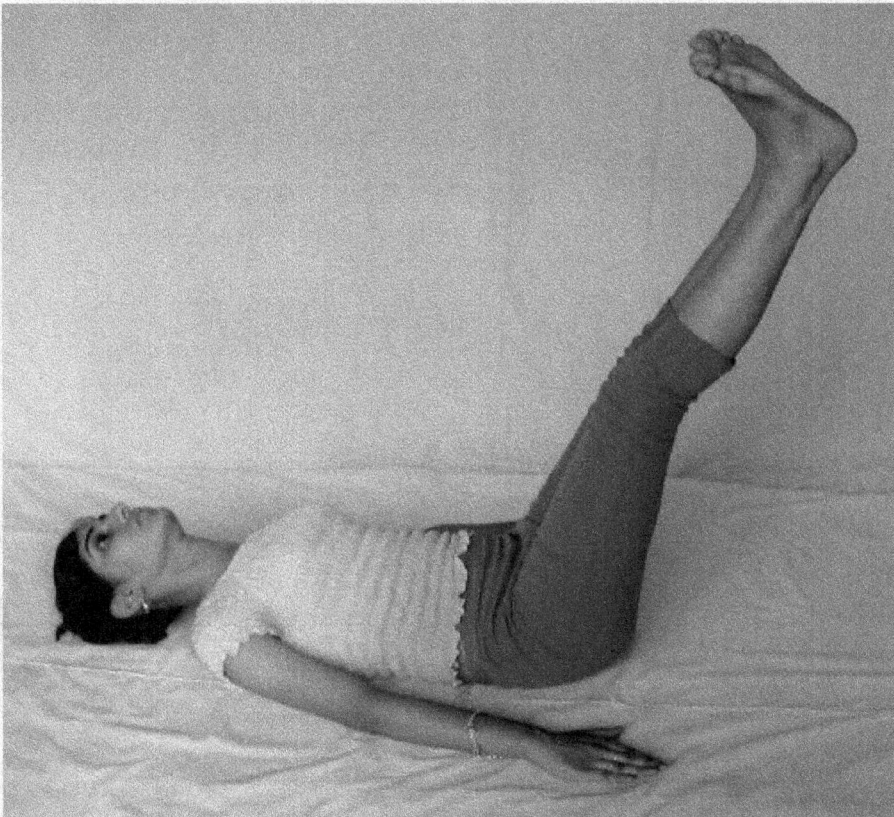

These asanas energise your abdominal muscles, internal organs of abdomen and pelvic joints. They are very efficient in reducing the excessive weight from abdomen. They are very good for blood circulation and for opening energy channels in the whole body. These asanas are recommended to cure sciatica pain.

Yogasana number 3

Paschimouttanasana (the forward stretching posture): Lie down on your back in a relaxed position with legs slightly apart from each other. Stretch your arms upwards and make sure that they are parallel to each other. The palms of your hands should face upwards. Lie like this for a little while and let yourself completely loose. Raise yourself from the lying position to a sitting position in such a way that while you are raising yourself, your head stays between your arms. From sitting position, bend forward in a similar manner until your hands touch your feet and your head is above your knees. Your knees should not bend.

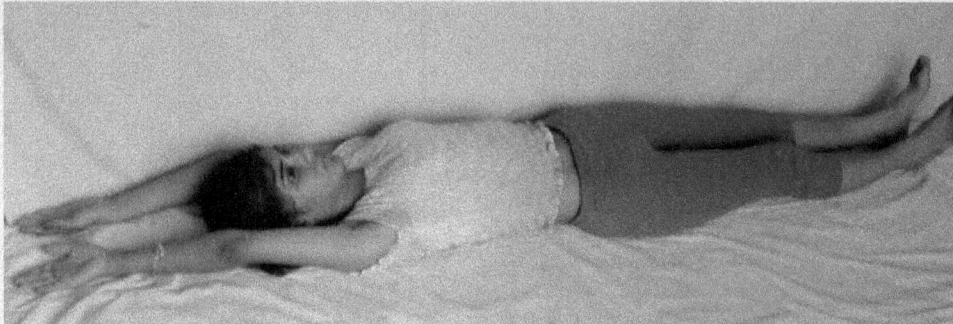

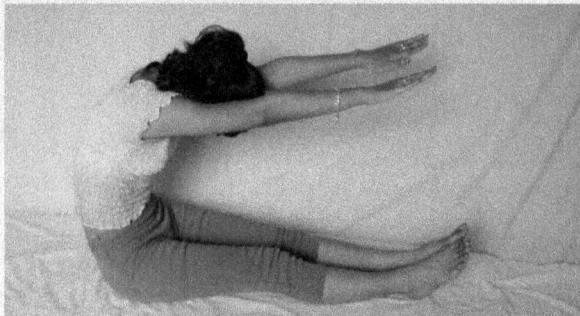

This posture helps you to acquire a straight and upright shoulder posture and open all the srotas of your body.

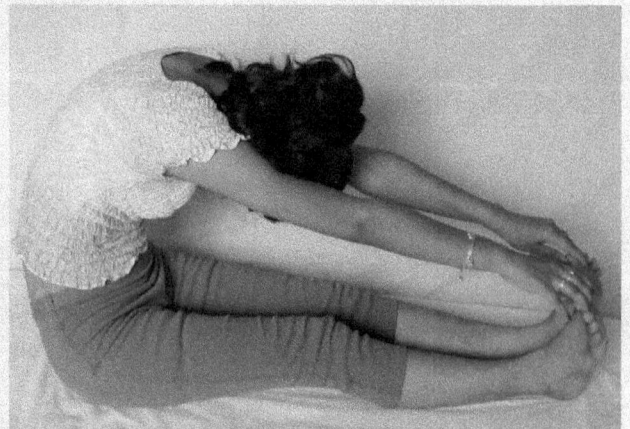

Yogasana number 4

Bhujangasana (Cobra posture): Lie down on your stomach with your chin on the floor and your bent arms and your palms touching the floor nearly at the level of your chest. Raise your head and chest gradually. Put your body pressure on your hands and bend your neck as far behind as you can without being uncomfortable. Your arms should be straight in this posture.

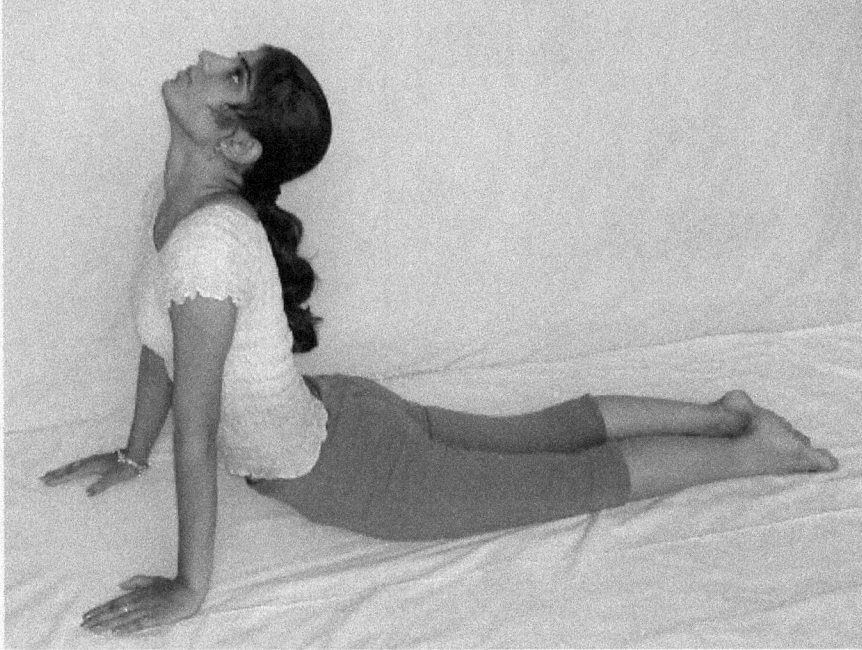

This is an excellent posture to make you strong and to give elasticity to your back. It opens energy channels in the chest and purifies lungs by pushing air in their profoundest parts. This asana also save you from wrinkles in your neck and from getting double chin.

Yogasana number 5

Halasana (Plough posture): Lie down on your back with your arms slightly away from your body and your feet joined together as you did in uttanapadasana when you raised both your legs. Raise your legs gradually and move them towards your head. The knees should not bend. Move your feet further and lower them to touch the ground above your head.
This is a wonderful asana to make your body supple internally as well as externally. This asana provides you a youthful vigour. It opens all the energy channels and purifies you by enhancing the blood flow.

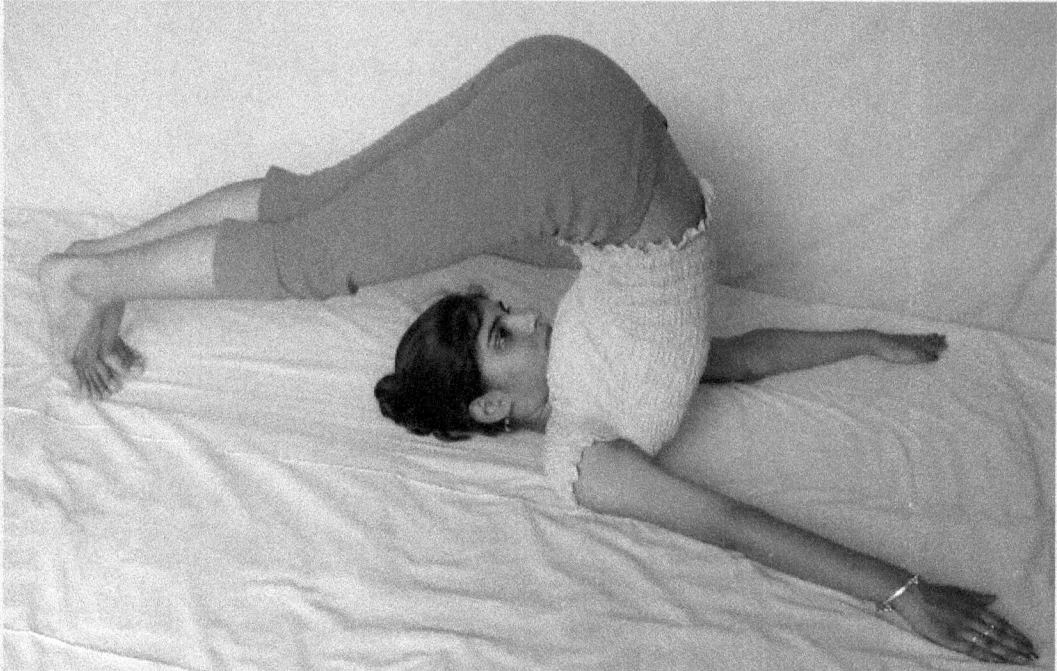

Yoganritya* or Yogic dance

Twenty-three years ago, I used some steps of classical Indian dance in my yoga class very spontaneously. The idea was very basic–to calm down people who came to me after work and were still under tension or excitation relating to the events of the day. Later, I wrote these steps in my first book on Yoga that was published in 1988. Ever since I have developed yoganritya as a form of relaxation and concentrating the mind on the body and have been teaching to my students.

The diverse forms of classical Indian dances are not merely the body movements with strict rules but are very transcendental and spiritual. Inspired by it, I have evolved the yoganritya or the yogic dance. I will write a separate book on this theme but I give you below some very basic steps of yoganritya and you will experience its wonder on your body and mind. If you practice it regularly, you will get a flexible body, enhanced mental concentration and shree.

* Copy right term

Step 1

Stand straight. Let yourself lose and take your torso slightly at the back to make a correct standing posture. Tap your left foot on the ground, then right and then left again and finally right. You have done 1,2,3,4 tapings like this. Continue the rhythm but this time, begin number 1 from 4. Your feet will tap in the following order: 1, 2, 3, 4; 4, 3, 2, 1; 1, 2, 3, 4; 4, 3, 2, 1.... and so on. Do it very slowly in the beginning and gradually make the rhythm faster.

Easy as it may sound, it is quite difficult to do it continuously for a few minutes. It needs your complete attention and the moment your thoughts are diverted, you will make a mistake. I have great fun with the students while doing this exercise. I check each one of them by looking at their feet and most of them make a mistake when I look at them. Their concentration is disturbed because I am looking at them. This makes them realise that for doing this step of yoganritya, their total attention is required.

Take care that your movement for tapping your foot is by bending slightly your knee. The upper part of the body stays relaxed. Some students make the mistake of moving their whole body when they tap their foot. Stay very relaxed, lift your foot about ten cm above the floor and tap your sole. Do these movements for several days until you can do very smoothly in a rhythmical manner. This step will be incorporated later with the hand movements.

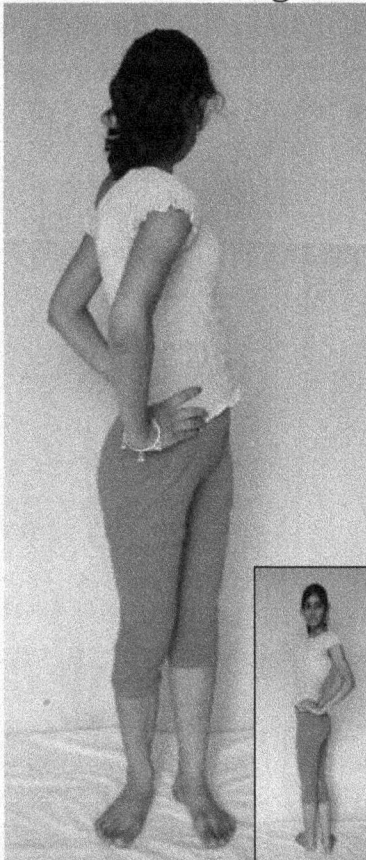

Step 2

Stand straight in the right posture as has been described above. Put your hands on your waste with fingers in front and thumb at the back. Move your waist very gently towards left by taking a turn of 180^0. It means that you can look at things at your back. Be careful that your neck does not move independently. The movement is only from the waist. Your feet also should not turn in this process. Come back to the original position in the same slow rhythm. Rest for few breaths and turn right with the same rhythm. Repeat the movements about 5 times.

Step 3

Step 2 is preparatory for step 3. Make the same movements with your waist but this time your arms are also involved. Make the movement from the waist in a similar manner as above to the left. Simultaneously, with the same rhythm as you move your waist towards left, go on lifting your right arm towards left in such a way that when your waist is at 180^0 angle, your arm is over your head. While you are reverting back your waist, revert back your arm by encircling it from the back in rhythm with your waist. Take a rest for few breaths and repeat the same by making waist movements towards right and moving your left arm this time. Repeat the movements about 5 times.

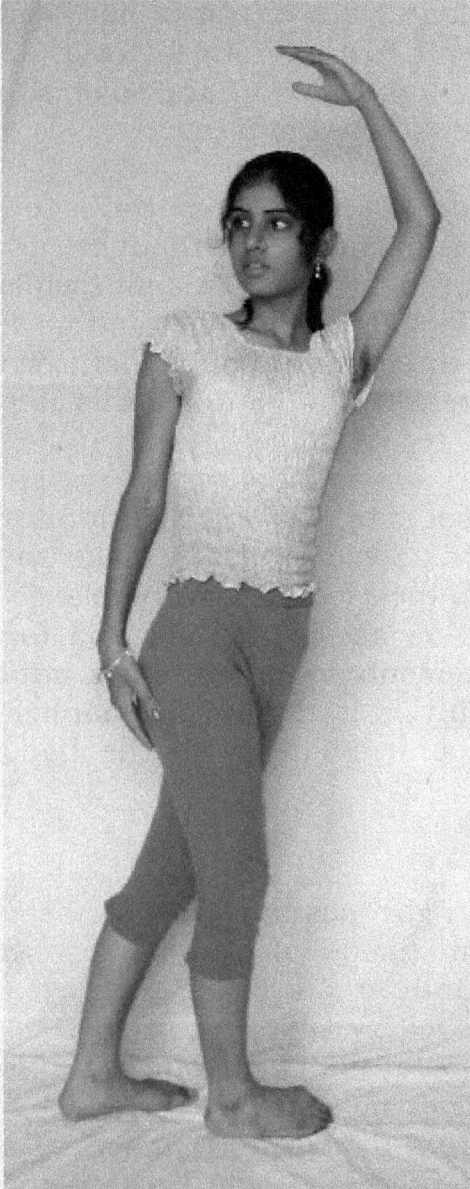

Step 4

In this step, you are going to repeat the step 3 in a spontaneous manner (not calculative) and are also going to involve your legs. Turn more than 180° by turning your feet along with your waist and make movement with your arm as above. However, keep your movements slow. You can do this step along with some music. Do this step for 2-3 minutes.

Step 5

This step includes hand and arm movements in rhythm with the step one. Repeat step one few times to make sure that you are doing it correctly. Then put both your hands face to face in front of your chest in such a manner that the index finger and thumb of each hand are touching each other and middle fingers of both the hands are face to face. Follow the sequence given below.

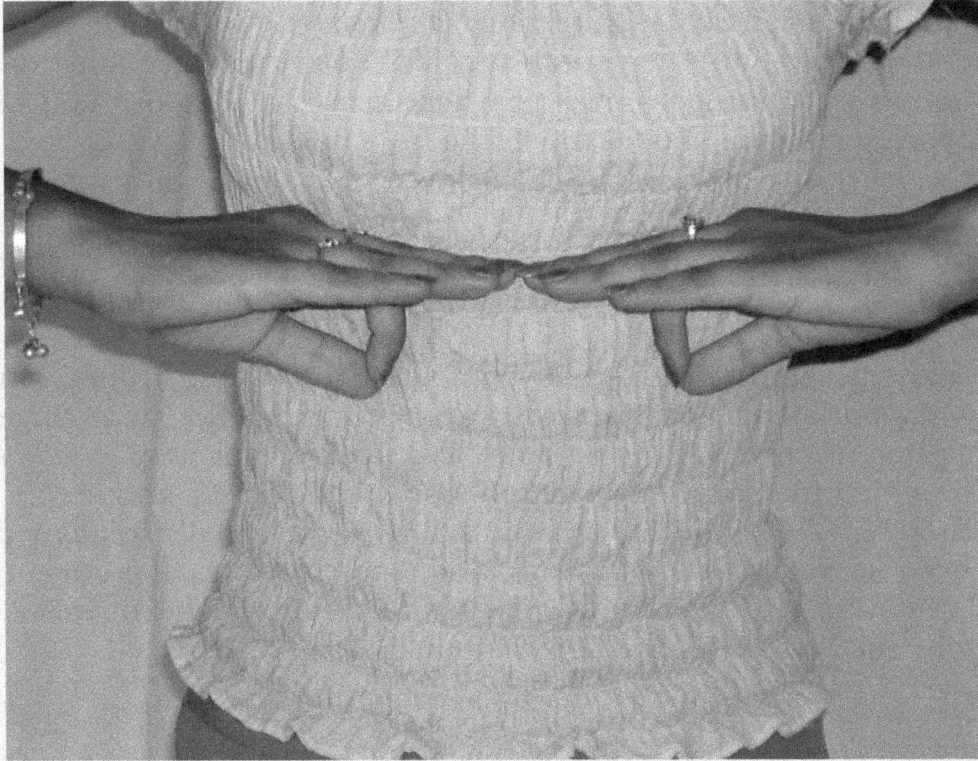

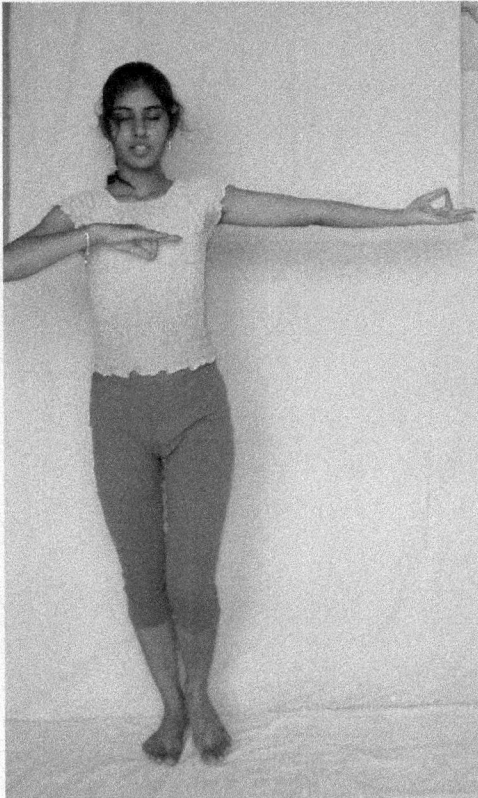
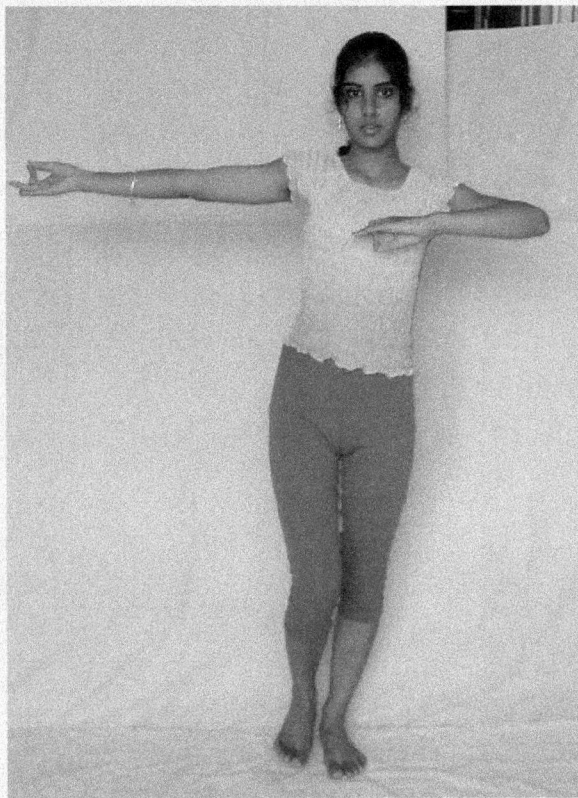

- Stamp your left foot again while extending out the left arm and your hands should have the thumb touching the ring finger this time.
- Stamp your right foot now, with right arm extended out and the thumbs of both the hands should touch the little finger.
- Stay in the above position with your arm and stamp your right foot again.
- Stamp the left foot and left arm should be extended out. Remember to touch the ring fingers of both the hands with their respective thumbs.

Continue in the same manner. Remember to coordinate the position of the fingers with your steps. For example, you are touching the small finger with the thumb at step number 4. You began in this position the step 1. The step 2 will involve touching the ring finger, step 3, the middle finger and step 4 the index finger. The step 1 begins from here again. You will need a regular practice to make these movements rhythmical and spontaneous. If your attention is diverted, each time, you will give a pause to think which finger should touch the thumb. That will break the flow of your movements.

7
Enhancing Beauty with Cosmic Bodies

Until now, I have described how you can work with your body to enhance your strength, charm, beauty and glamour. All these put together are Shree and rupa in you. The purpose of all these practices is to bring out the sunshine and radiance which lies hidden in each one of us. What hides that inner light? What hinders its path? Imbalance at physical or mental level or both together makes a cover of darkness around our inner light. With all your efforts until now, you have purified yourself, open the srotas or energy channels of the body and have paved way to be in harmony with the rest of the cosmos. Once you are in harmony within yourself and with your immediate surroundings, try to enhance your energy further by interacting with cosmic bodies. In fact, there is tremendous energy around us, but we do not take advantage of it. Urban folks around the world have no relationship with their cosmic surroundings. Many of them are quite unaware of different phases of the moon. Those who work in closed spaces with artificial light and air-conditioning have also no relationship with the light of the day, the sun and the subtle changes in the climate.

Given below are some simple methods which you may use to enhance your radiance.

Relationship of the sun to aging

Sun defines time as a day is defined with the rising and setting of the sun. The days turn into weeks and weeks into months and that is how the years go by and so is our life. Change is the inherent nature of time. Thus, each day brings some change in our existence at diverse levels. We go through various phases of life and degenerative changes with aging are the on going process of nature. Our aim should be to minimize this degeneration. In the Vedic tradition, a great emphasis is laid on the sun worship and daily prayers to the sun. I have incorporated one such prayer from the Rig Veda in my Ayurvedic daily routine that I have described in my books. That is a prayer to the sun that is done upon getting up in the morning, asking for blessing for a long and healthy life, protection of all the five senses and for seeing many-many days like this in future.

Assimilating shree from the sun

The sun is the radiance of our cosmos. The element sun is within us in the form of pitta energy. At a subtle level, sattva is our inner light. Sattva is our shree. Try to evoke a relationship with the sun to enhance your inner light. Do the following to make yourself conscious about the cosmic energy of the sun and develop a relationship with this powerful cosmic body.

I suggest that you think of the sun at least two times a day, at the time of the sunrise or immediately upon getting up, and at the time of the sunset. Wherever you are and whatever you are doing, time yourself to the sun twice a day. In the Vedic tradition, it is believed that there is a special energy in the atmosphere at the time of sunrise and sunset. Agnihotra Yagya, which was originally to promote agriculture, was done at these timings. In any case, I suggest that you do your own ritual with the sun in your own simple way. Pray at the time of the sunrise and the sunset for giving you a little bit from his abundance shree (radiance).

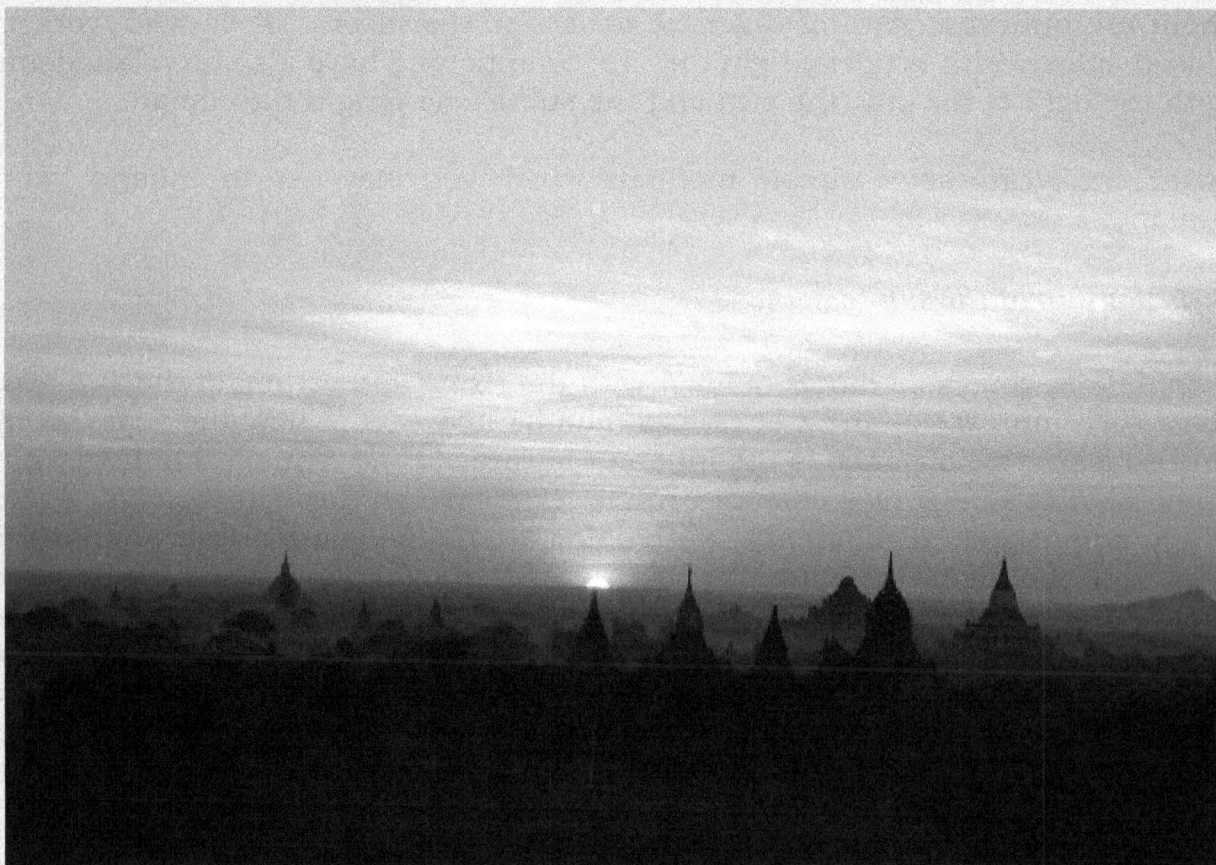

If you have tamasic feeling like jealousy, anger, revenge, greed, etc., pray to the abundance shree of the sun to get rid of them. The powerful sun's energy can help you get rid of the darkness in your mind. The divine light of the sun can enlighten your inner being and can give you beauty, goodness and strength.

In the Vedic tradition, Gayatri mantra is recited to get blessings and energy from the sun. It is a very beautiful and powerful mantra and I suggest that you recite it regularly to see its effect. I give below the transcription of the original Sanskrit mantra from the Rig Veda, its literal as well as poetic translation.

Gayatri Mantra

Om bhur-bhuvh svah
Tat savitru-varenyam
Bhargo devasya dhimahi
Dhiyo yo nh prachodhayat.

Literal translation:

In the entire cosmos at physical, astral and celestial planes
That adorable radiating One
We meditate on the splendour of the remover of ignorance
Who promotes intellect and enlightens us.

Poetic translation:

Adorable and splendid in the entire cosmos,
we meditate on the glory of That shinning One,
remover of all ignorance,
who promotes intellect and enlightens us.

Assimilating wisdom and charm from the moon

Moon influences our mind. Moon is the symbol of wisdom. In the Vedic tradition, it is believed that moon is related to water element and provides healing energy called soma to the medicinal plants Assimilate moon's soma by developing a contact with it. Always remember the day of the ascending and descending moon. Think of the moon before going to bed each night and pray to it to give you mental stability and strength. Try to look at the moon as much as possible.

Full moon is the symbol of beauty and perfection. Always remember to pay homage to the moon on the day of its full glory. Seek blessings for good health and attractive appearance from the moon. Full moon has a tremendous enchanting energy. For romance and for attracting attention of someone of the opposite sex, specifically pray to the moon on the full moon day.

Moon has also cooling and peaceful energy and pray to the full moon to pacify you if you have an aggravated and easily irritable character.

Learning to be flexible from water

Water is one of the five elements that constitute our body. Everything is functional because of water because in the solid form, the body cannot exist. You should assimilate from water the energy of fluidity and flexibility. In fact, persons who are very tough and hard and want to do things in a mechanical way, acquire a very hard expression on their faces. Massage, anointing and all the other treatments described earlier cannot help them to get rid of the hard expression which makes them quite unattractive. A mechanical and stiff attitude for doing things or dealing with life events affects your srotas or energy channels. It also gives rise to mental blockades and an unattractive look.

It is interesting that when a woman happens to have this kind of hard expression that I have described above, she is designated as being 'manly' or 'masculine'. I do not agree with this description that this kind of expression makes a woman look unlike a woman. It is simply unpleasant and unattractive. A hard expression takes away the beauty and charm from any human being– be it a man, woman or child. Imagine a so-called 'masculine' looking woman with a man's body. You still would not find that face attractive. It is not a secret that most women like men with tender expressions and tender behaviour. In fact, the results of my two decades research on men-women relationships and sexuality show that most women in the world complain about the lack of tenderness in their men. Thus, I suggest strongly that all of you try to assimilate this soft energy from water.

You can do concentration practices on water near a water source like river, lake or sea. Alternatively, you can concentrate on element water each morning when you take your bath or shower. Concentrate on the movements and the flow of water. Admire its beauty and cleansing capabilities. Think of the tenderness of water when it touches your body. Pray to the flowing water to bless you with flexibility, tender heart and loving face expression.

Assimilate vastness from the sky

Element ether or space is one of the five elements which form our body. Without space, nothing can exist. The element wind exists in space. Existence of element fire is dependent on air and space both. Water has all the previous three elements. And earth is complete with the existence of all the five elements in it.

Concentrate on the beauty and vastness of the sky on a clear day or on a clear summer night. Assimilate this vastness with your eyes and then close your eyes to concentrate all your thoughts on the image you have had in your mind. If your thoughts begin to wander, open your eyes again and assimilate the vastness and try to meditate again.

Pray to the sky to bless you with grandeur and charm. Seek blessings to attain a large heart with forgiveness and kindness. Assimilate the peaceful atmosphere in you and get rid of your ego and the problems related to it. Under this vast space, there are millions of people who have even worse problems than you have. After these thoughts, try to meditate again on the vastness and assimilate its energy.

Assimilating grandeur, strength, beauty and longevity of banyan tree

Deep rooted and long-life trees like banyan or peepal or kuchala (*Nux vomica*) are a symbol of longevity and wisdom in Vedic tradition. They are considered as holy and small temple icons are built under these trees. They are worshiped for long life, health and fulfilment of other wishes. They are symbolic of the abundance energy of the element earth. To assimilate grandeur, beauty and energy for long life, I suggest that you concentrate on one of these trees.

Choose one of the beautiful big trees in your vicinity and find time once a week to go close to it and touch its stem. Take deep breaths from its energetic air and pray to it to bless you with its grandeur, beauty and longevity. Wish for yourself the strength of this tree. A deep-rooted tree stays strong in face of storms and winds and does not fall. Put your both hands on the stem and touch it also with your forehead in reverence for the element earth.

111

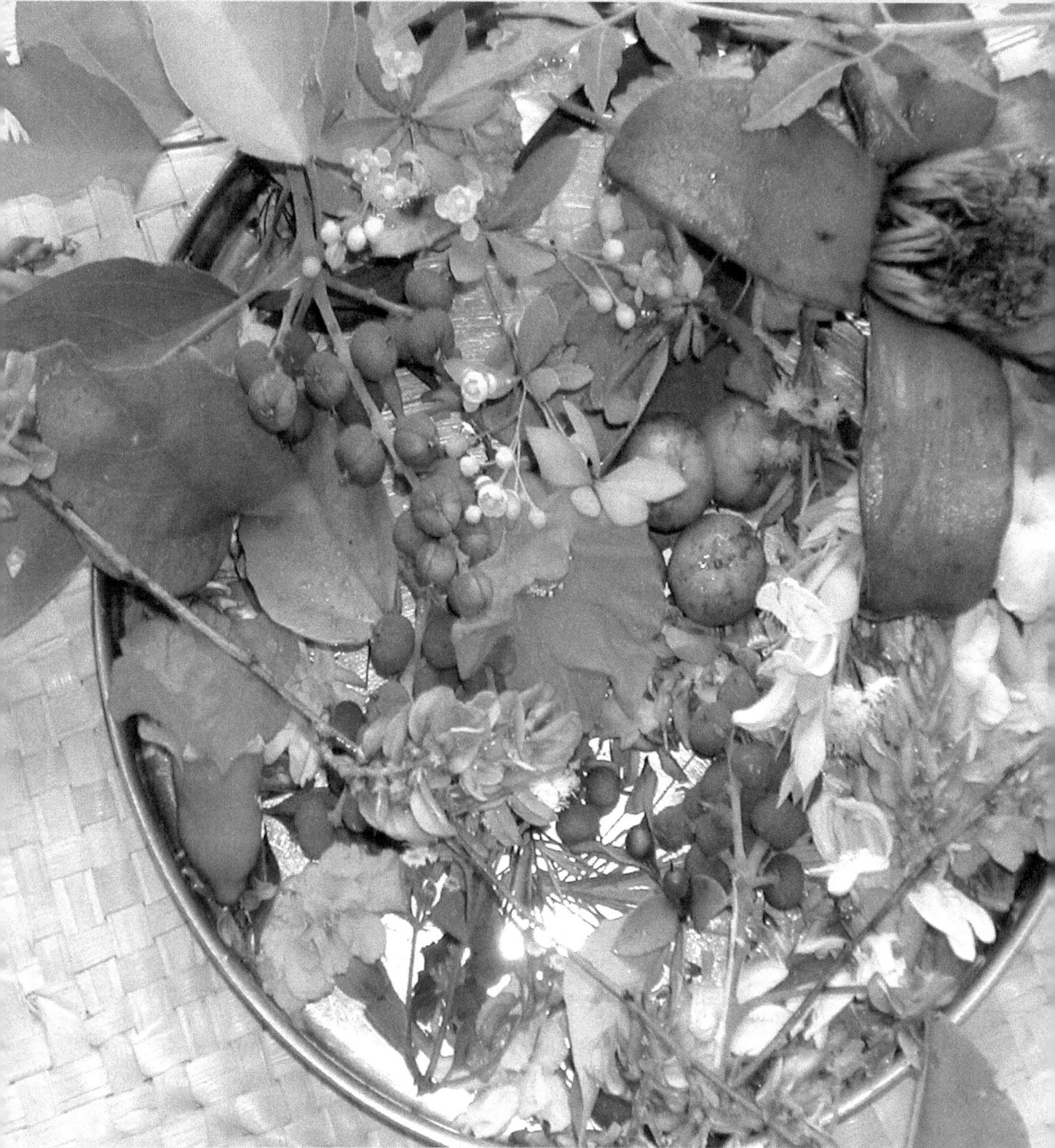

8

Description of Products mentioned in this Book

I have given here the description of various products mentioned in this book in an alphabetical order. May be some of you already know about many of these products. These products are available on the Indian shops or oriental shops abroad. Some of them can also be bought from the Health Stores or from seed shops. I have specified in each case. In case something is not available on Indian shops, you can request the owner to get it for you.

It is possible that the shop owners do not know the German or English names. Besides that, some times there are misnomers used for certain products. To avoid getting a wrong product, it is important that you take the book with you and show the Hindi or North Indian name mentioned below. The products for which no English or German names are available (like ajwain), I have used the Hindi name and given the Latin name along side.

Ajwain

Latin name of ajwain is *Trichyspermum ammi.* Ajwain seeds are very tiny, light brown in colour; nearly heart shaped and have lines on their surface. Ajwain smells similar to thyme because they both have etheric oil called Thymene. Outside the Indian continent, it is available in Indian shops.

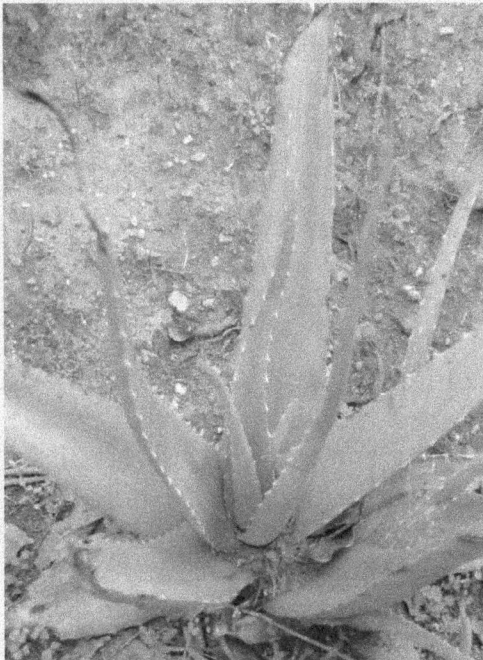

Aloe vera

This small cactus plant is called *Aloe vera* in *Latin* and Kumari or ghee Kumari in Hindi. The thick succulent leaves of this cactus have a ghee like substance and that is the reason for its name. The plant is available all over India in the nurseries and you can grow it in your garden in a big pot. You can also bring one leaf and put it in a pot. It propagates very fast. Do not give too much water to it. In cold countries, put the plant indoors in winter. I recommend that you get at least one plant of Aloe and then make several plants out of it. It is a very useful plant to have at home as the ghee or the viscous substance inside its leaves is wonderful for a wound, cut, skin eruption or rough skin, besides its use for a mask as described earlier in this book.

Chickpea flour (besan)

Basin (North Indian, Hindi name) is not the flour of big white chickpeas which most of you are familiar with. For making basin, a smaller and darker variety of chickpeas called black gram (kalachana in Hindi, literally meaning black chickpea) is used. These chickpeas are brown in colour and about 30% smaller that the other chickpeas most of you know. The flour is made after removing the husk.

Chickpea flour (rough)

Same grain is used as described above for besan but this flour is made without removing the husk. It is also not ground so fine.

Cress seeds

Cress or Garden cress in Latin is called *Lepidium sativum*. It is called Chandrashoor in Sanskrit; Chansoor and Halim are some other North Indian names. Cress seeds are easily available also in Europe and America but in seed shops, as the leaves of cress are eaten as a salad. In India, it is cultivated for fodder for horses[*], whereas the seeds are used in medicine.

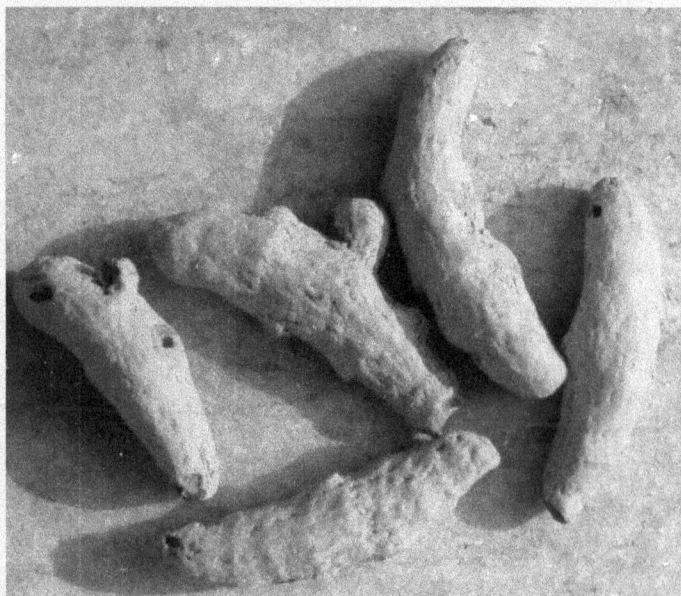

Curcuma (haldi)

Everybody in the world knows about curcuma or turmeric. Mostly it is sold in powder form. In the monsoon season, the fresh curcuma is also available. It is a root like ginger with bright yellow colour. In India, many people buy dried roots and get the powder made in order to be sure that it is not older than a year. If you buy powdered curcuma abroad, make sure that the packing is not more than six months old. Generally in

[*] Horse is a symbol for health and strength in Ayurveda. Black gram as well as cress are horse foods and evidently strength-promoting for human beings.

Indian stores abroad, it is always fresh as they sell a lot.

Chiraunji

It is a nut from a big tree that grows wild and is also cultivated in Central India. I did not find any English name for it but in Latin it is called *Buchanania lanzan*. Chiraunji nuts are used in food in India and are also used in Ayurvedic remedies of beauty and brain. It strengthens the nerves besides the beauty applications that you have learnt in this book.

Coconut oil

Coconut oil is also called coconut fat as it begins to solidify at temperatures lower than 25^0 C. The oil is extracted from dried coconuts. It is easily available abroad on Indian shops as well as on health food stores. Do not go in for coconut oil from Ayurvedic companies. Firstly they make it expensive; secondly sometimes I found it mixed with some other fat. Go in for simple coconut oil that people in South India use for cooking. What ghee in North is, coconut oil is in the south. I found the brand name *Parachute* has very good quality and is also easily available at Indian shops abroad.

Do not melt all the coconut oil you have each time. Take smaller quantity in another bottle or a metal bowl. With frequent melting, sometimes the oil starts smelling unpleasant.

Liquorice

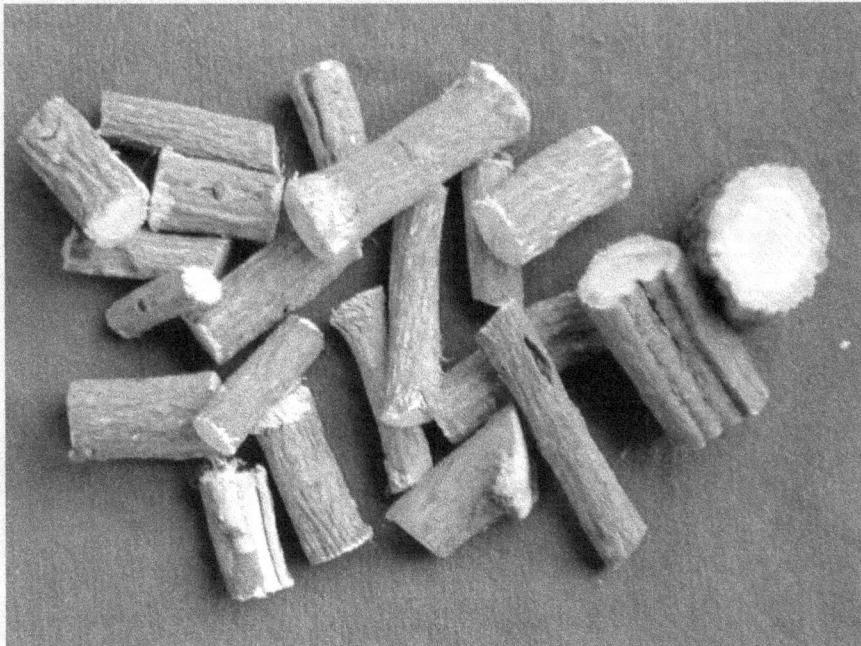

It is a root. It is fifty times more sweet than the sugar. In many countries, candies are made from it. Do not buy already powdered liquorice. You can grind it in a coffee grinder which should be exclusively devoted to herbs and spices. If the roots are big, crush them a little with the stone or metal grinder before putting them into the coffee grinder for powdering them. Make the fine powder as has been described above.

Orange peels

Save the peels from organically grown oranges. Take oranges or mandarins with fine skin, cut the peels into small pieces and dry them. Grind and make fine powder as described above.

Mustard oil

In India, mustard oil is very common as it is also used in cooking. In the West, mustard oil can be bought at the Indian stores. Make sure when you buy mustard or sesame oils that these are not refined and are cold pressed. Once I bought a bottle of sesame oil in a German store and this oil had no flavour at all. It was highly refined oil imported from China. This kind of product has no effective qualities of the original natural product you are meant to use.

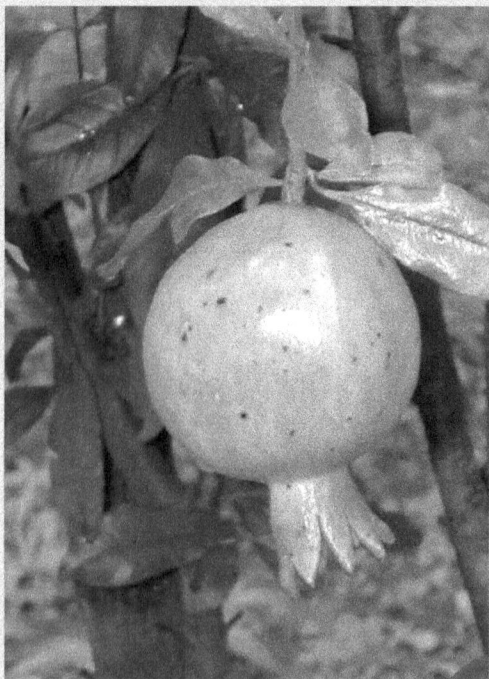

Pomegranate peels

Pomegranate peel has many medicinal qualities and in dried and powdered form it is used for the care of teeth, in brain rejuvenating products as well as for skin treatment. Wash the peels and cut them into small pieces so that they are easy to make a powder after drying.

Rock salt

Rock salt is called sendha namak in Hindi. It has pink-peach colour. It is available on the Indian stores abroad in powdered form. There is also a dark variety of rock salt which is called kala namak or black salt.

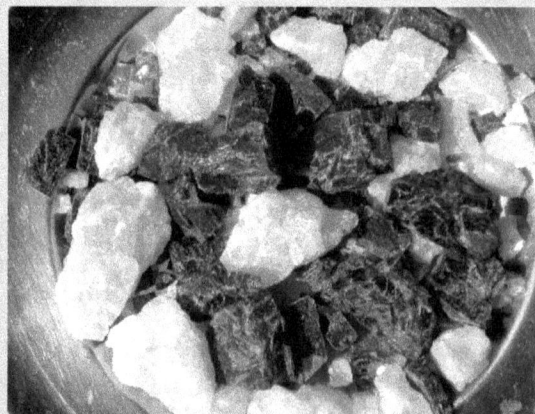

This variety has ammonia salts and smells very strong. Use preferably the pure sendha namak.

Sandalwood paste

Little pieces of sandalwood are available for making paste. The paste is made by rubbing sandalwood on the stone with flat surface. Wet the stone and then put about ½ teaspoon of water on it. Start rubbing the sandalwood on it by applying pressure. Add few more drops of water. You will see that the paste is made. Put this paste in a small bowl and make more paste the same way. Accumulate the paste until you have the desired quantity.

Sandalwood paste can also be obtained from sandalwood powder. Add water into the powder to make a thick paste. Whip well and add a little more water. Pass this paste through muslin cloth and squeeze out the fine sandalwood paste. You can use the paste as such without passing it through muslin cloth but it is very rough and does not feel good on the skin.

There exists also red sandalwood which is used for beauty. But this is not perfumed like the other sandalwood. It is also used for beautification and for temple ceremonies. It is Ayurvedic function is like the other sandalwood as it is also cold in its properties.

Sesame paste

Sesame paste can be made by crushing the sesame seeds in a grinder. This paste is also available in the Turkish or Middle Eastern shops abroad. It is called Tahini.

Shirish powder

Shirish is a mimosa family tree and is called *Albizzia lebbeck* in Latin. It is a very big, wild tree that grows all over India except in the high mountains. Seeds are in pods and each pod has 6 to 10 seeds. The pods dry on the trees and fall down in the month of February and March. Take the seeds out from the pods and dry for another two to three days in the sun. Make powder with a grinder and then a fine powder as described above.

Combs of natural substances

Combs are available in wood, sandalwood and many other natural products. In the former times, they were also available in ivory and horn. Thanks to the Animal Protection groups that this trade is almost finished. If possible, get a wooden comb rather than a plastic. Head is the coolest part of the body and plastic generates heat. Iron or other metal combs are also available. They are also good for massaging the head. They are particularly good if your head remains unusually warm.

Fine powder

To obtain a fine powder from a substance, you have to make powder with the grinder, then pass it through a fine strainer and finally pass it through a muslin cloth. Stretch a muslin cloth on a small pot and put a rubber band around it to hold it. Put some powder on the cloth and move it with a spoon. The fine powder will accumulate underneath.

Healing earth

Healing earth is also called Multani mitti in north India. It is named after the area from where it came in the past. Multan is a part of Pakistan now. It is a fine, yellow coloured earth. It is available also on Health stores in Europe and America. Generally it is called healing earth.

AUM SHANTI

About the Author

After a doctorate degree in reproduction biology in India, Dr. Verma studied Neurobiology in Paris University and obtained a second doctorate. She pursued advanced research at the National Institutes of Health, Bethesda (USA) and the Max-Planck Institute in Freiburg, Germany. At the peak of her career in medical research in a pharmaceutical company in Germany, she realised that the modern approach to health care is basically fragmented and non-holistic. Besides, we are directing all our efforts and resources to cure disease rather than maintaining health. In response, Dr. Verma founded The New Way Health Organisation (NOW) in 1986 to spread the message of holistic living, preventive methods for health care and to promote the use of mild medicine and various self-help therapeutic measures.

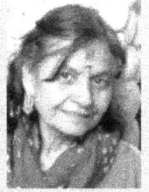

Dr. Verma grew up with a strong familial tradition of Ayurveda with a grandmother who had enormous Ayurvedic wisdom and was a gifted healer. She has studied Ayurveda in the traditional Guru-shishya style with Acharya Priya Vrat Sharma of the Benares Hindu University for 23 years.

Dr. Verma is an ardent researcher and is working hard to compile the living tradition of Ayurveda and spread it in the world through her books. She has published 23 books on yoga, Ayurveda, Women and Companionship. The books are published in various languages of the world. Besides, she has published numerous scientific articles. Several other books are in preparation. She lectures extensively, teaches in Europe for several months a year, trains students at her two centres in India and gives radio and television programmes. First film on Ayurveda was made by German television on Dr. Verma and was shown in 100 countries in 130 languages.

Dr. Verma has founded Charaka School of Ayurveda to train interested people with genuine Ayurvedic education so that they can further impart the knowledge of Ayurvedic way of life and save people from becoming a victim of charlatanry in Ayurveda. Dr. Verma is doing several research projects on medicinal plants and their combination in the form of remedies. She is the founder and chairperson of *The Ayurveda Health Organisation*, which is a charitable trust for distributing and promoting Ayurvedic remedies and yoga therapy in rural areas of India. She does regular lectures and workshops for school children in the rural and remote areas of the Himalayas to promote wisdom of traditional science and medicine. Dr. Verma gives seminars, lectures and teaches in the *Charaka School of Ayurveda* with guru-shishya tradition.

Dr Verma speaks Hindi, Punjabi, French, German and English and she has knowledge of Sanskrit.

Author's Publications

1. *Patanjali's Yoga Sutra: A Scientific Exposition* (Published in English, Hindi and German).
2. *Ayurveda for Inner Harmony: Nutrition, Sexual Energy and Healing* (Published in English, German, Italian, French, Romanian and Hindi).
3. *Ayurveda a Way of Life* (Published in English, German, Italian, French, Spanish, Czech, Greek, Portuguese and Hindi).
4. *The Kamasutra for Women* (Published in English [America and India], German, French, Dutch, Romanian, Italian, Portuguese, Hindi and Malayalam).
5. *Stress-free Work with Yoga and Ayurveda* (Published in German, English [America and India] and Hindi).
6. *Patanjali and Ayurvedic Yoga* (Published in English, German and Hindi).
7. *Programming Your Life with Ayurveda* (Published in German, French, Slovenian, English and Czech).
8. *Ayurvedic Food Culture and Recipes* (Published in English, Czech, German and Hindi).
9. *Yoga: A Natural Way of Being* (Published in English, German, French, Italian and Hindi).
10. *Companionship and Sexuality (Based on Ayurveda and the Hindu tradition)* (Published in English and German).
11. *Natural Glamour: The Ayurveda Beauty Book* (Published in German, Spanish and English)
12. *Losing and Maintaining Weight with Ayurveda and Yoga* (Published in English, Slovenian and German).
13. *The Timeless Wisdom of Ayurveda: A Scientific Exposition* (Published in English and German)
14. *Prakriti and Pulse: The Two Mysteries of Ayurveda* (Published in German)
15. *Good Food for Dogs: Vegetarian nourishment based on Ayurvedic wisdom* (Published in German and English)
16. *Diet for Losing Weight* (published in German and English)
17. *Aum: The Infinite Energy* (Published in German and English)
18. *Pulse Diagnose in Chinese and Ayurvedic Medicine* (co-author for TCM Dr. Florian Ploberger) (published in German)
19. *Shiva's Secrets for Health and Longevity* (published in German and English)
20. *Healing Hands: The Ayurvedic Massage workbook* (in press)
21. *Prevention of Dementia* (published in German and English)
22. *Ayurveda for Dogs* (published in German)
23. *Numerology: Based on the Vedic Tradition* (published in English and Slovenian)

The Charaka School of Ayurveda and Patanjali Yogadarshana Society (Himalayan Centre)

The Charka School of Ayurveda (CSA) has been founded by Dr. Vinod Verma to spread the genuine classical tradition as well as the living tradition of Ayurveda in the world for promoting healthy living and preventing ailments. Its aim is to teach people a healthy lifestyle which enhances immunity and vitality and enables them to live a life with optimum level of energy. For minor ailments, people should be capable of using home remedies, appropriate physical and mental exercises and nutrition.

CSA aims to bring genuine and practical aspects of Ayurveda to people and save them from Americanised and Europeanised distorted versions of Ayurveda and other forms of charlatanry that do more harm than good.

To achieve this purpose, CSA organises to train students in Europe who can further spread the message of Ayurvedic lifestyle and help people with genuine massages, purification practices, nutrition and other practical aspects of Ayurveda. The school is in association with the most learned persons of Ayurveda in India and several exclusive persons involved in health education in Europe.

The object of Patanjali Yogadarshana Society is to spread the message of Patanjali in the world. The wisdom of the Yoga Sutras is not only beneficial for the yogis but also for our day-to-day normal life. Its aim is to enhance *sattva* or the inner stillness and peace in the world as well as in the individual minds. With years of research on Yoga and Ayurveda, Dr. Verma has founded the Ayurvedic Yoga and has written a book on the subject.

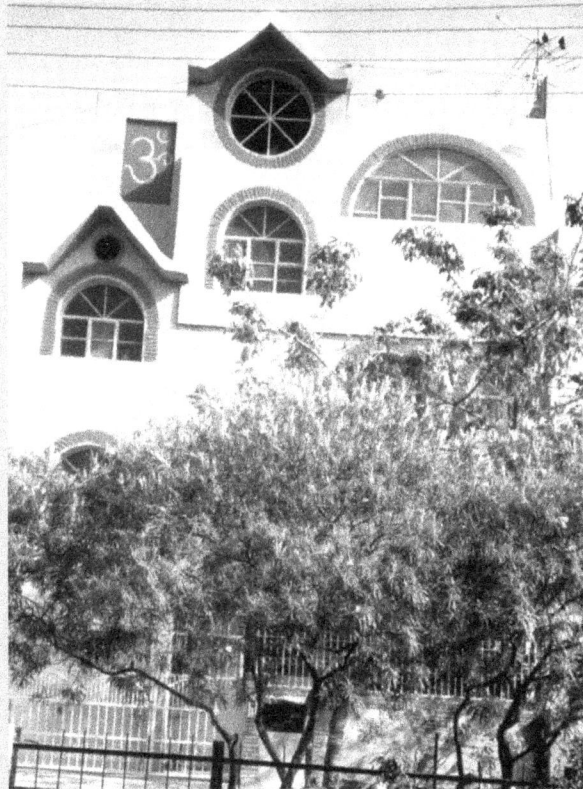

Noida Centre

Himalayan Centre

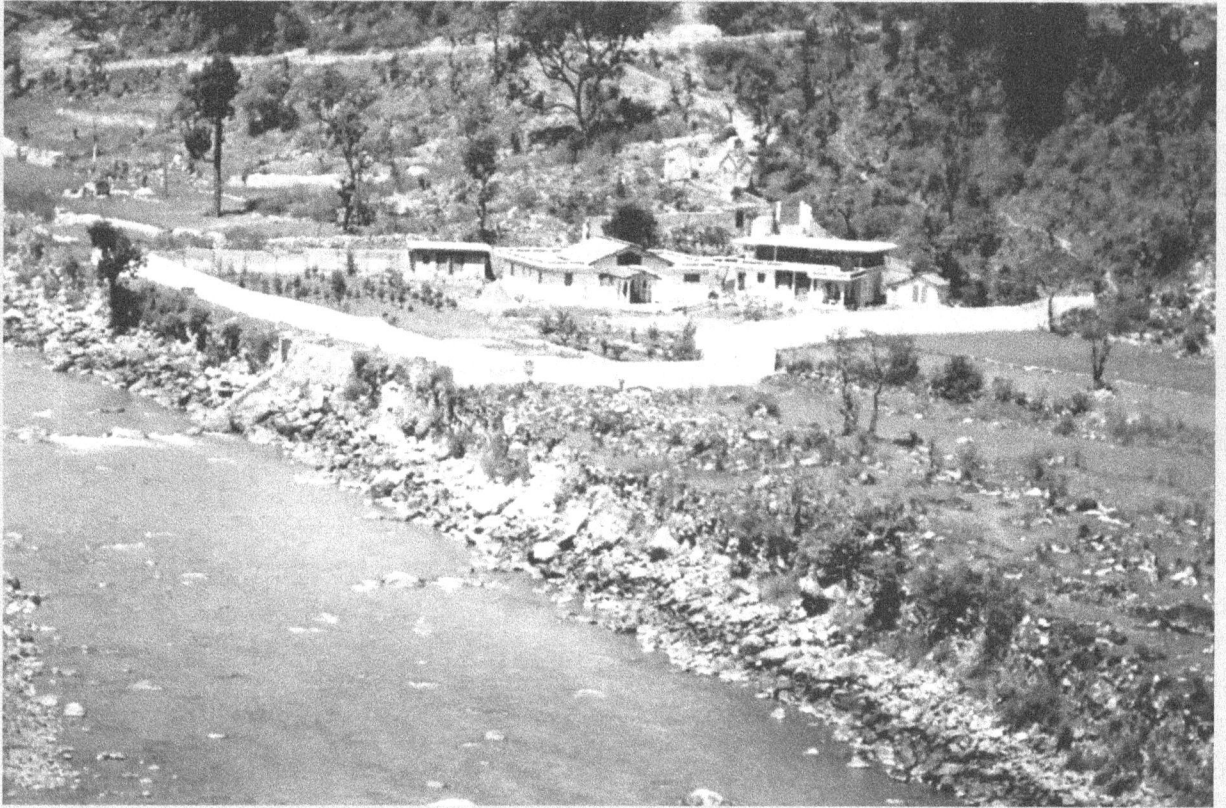

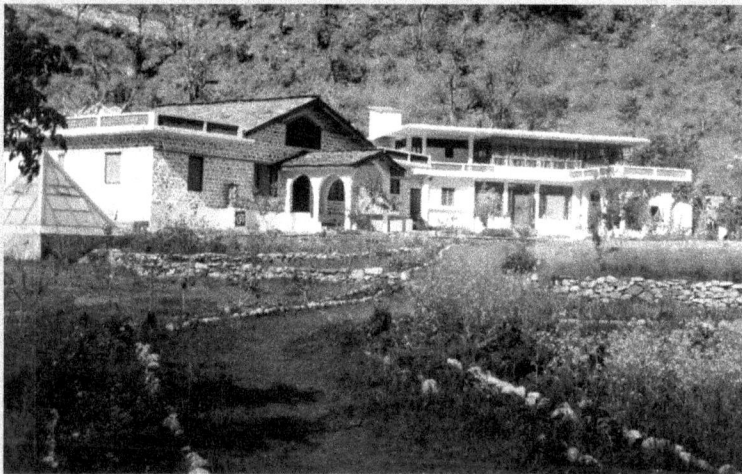

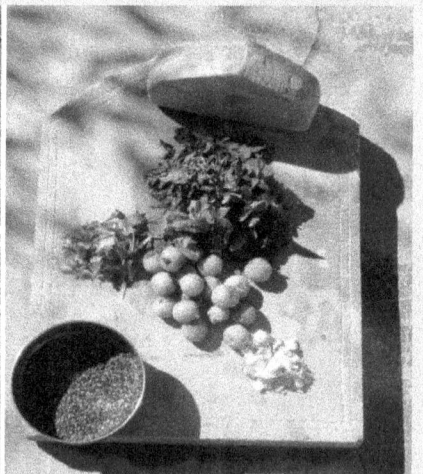

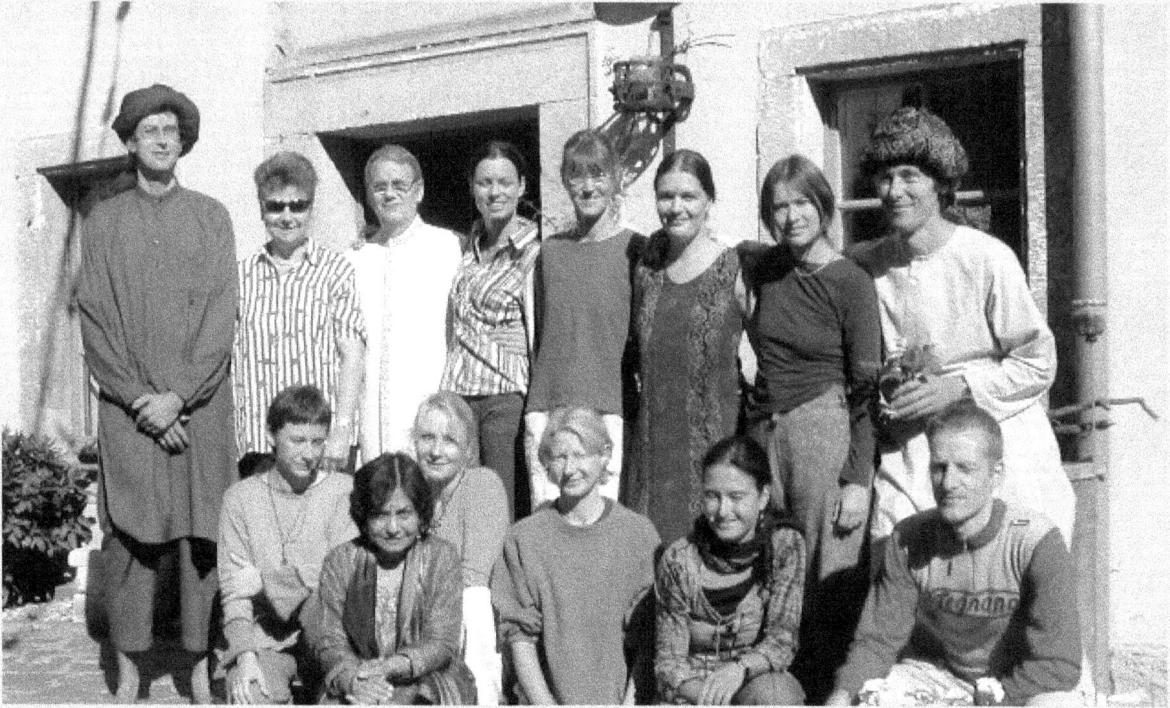

Lectures, Seminars and Training Programmes

To get detailed information on the Charaka School of Ayurveda as well as our other programmes in India and Europe, visit our website or email us to the following addresses:

The New Way Health Organisation .NOW.
A-130, Sector 26, Noida 201301, U.P., India
Tel. 0091 (0)120 2527820 or (0) 9873704205 or (0)9412224820
Email: ayurvedavv@yahoo.com or ayurvedavv@gmail.com
Website: www.ayurvedavv.com

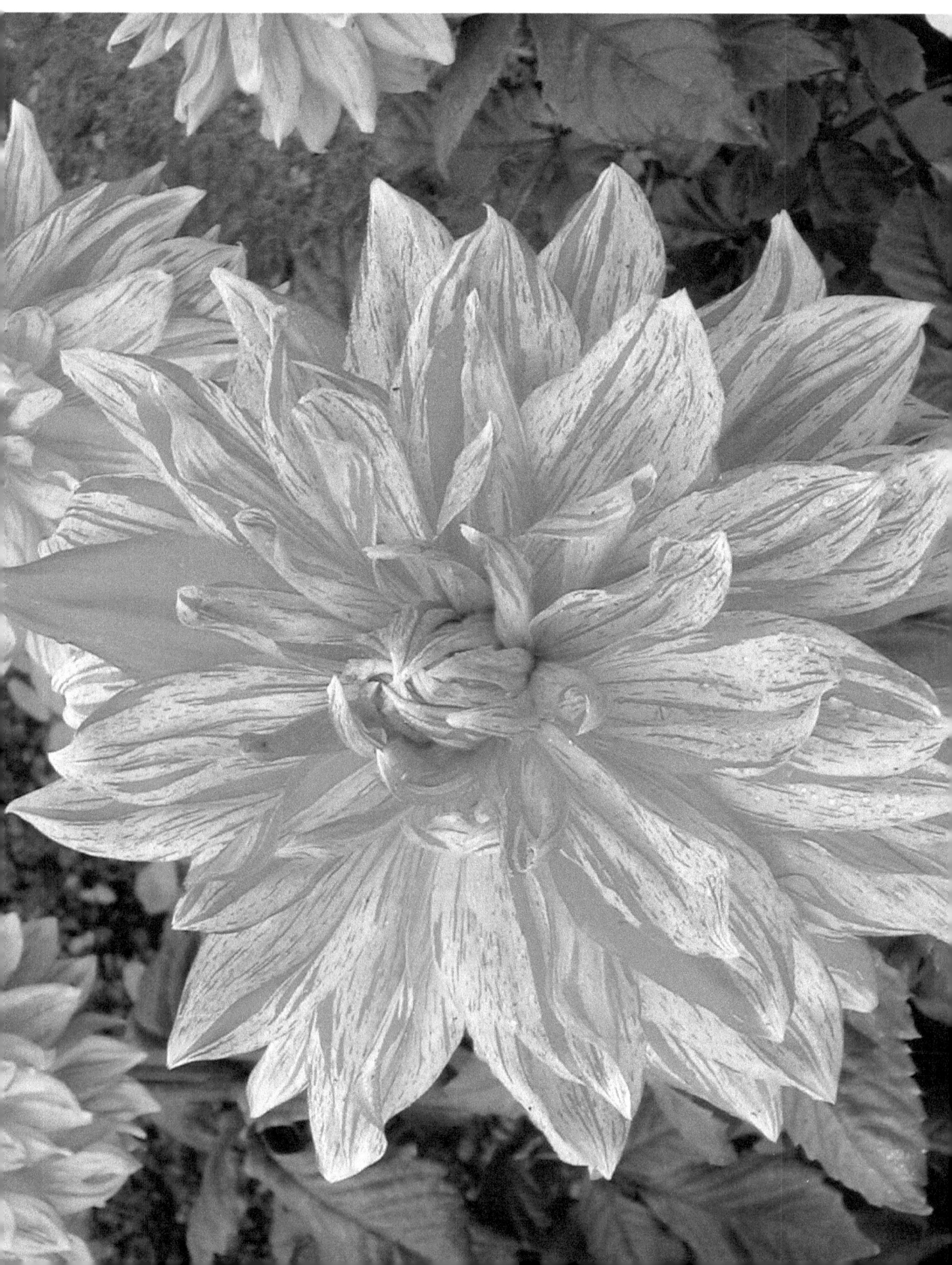

www.ingramcontent.com/pod-product-compliance
Lightning Source LLC
Chambersburg PA
CBHW081408270326
41931CB00016B/3419